## Praise f

## CALM YOUR



'[Calm Your Gut] *brings us back into connection with one of our most sacred events – eating food. This is one of the most powerful experiences in our day as, well beyond the simple provision of nutrients, the foods we choose to consume gift us an intense array of information that influences not only our metabolism and that of our gut microbes, but the expression of our DNA as well. It's time we embrace the profound nature of this seemingly mundane event and [this book] serves as your guide.'*

DR DAVID PERLMUTTER, #1 *NEW YORK TIMES* BESTSELLING AUTHOR OF *GRAIN BRAIN* AND *BRAIN WASH*

*'Cara Wheatley-McGrain puts the heart into the science of the human microbiome. Warm, helpful, comprehensible, practical and scientifically accurate, I would recommend this book to anyone who wants a wise and resourceful companion on their journey to true gut health.'*

SHANN NIX JONES, DIRECTOR OF CHUCKLING GOAT AND BESTSELLING AUTHOR OF *THE KEFIR SOLUTION*

'[Calm Your Gut] *will transform the gut of anyone who reads it. It's a refreshing take on being compassionate and loving your gut so much that your life and gut change naturally and organically. This book is just as fascinating as our digestive system! I recommend this book to anyone who struggles with gut issues including bloating, IBS, IBD, Crohn's disease, and even acne and psoriasis. If you want to become the architect of your own gut and health you will be glad you spent the time reading this book!'*

LIANA WERNER-GRAY, NUTRITIONIST AND BESTSELLING AUTHOR OF *THE EARTH DIET*

*'A fascinating and insightful book. Cara not only teaches us why gut health is so vitally important for mental and physical health, but she compassionately guides us through a diverse range of helpful strategies for improving our gut health and inspires us to take control of our health.'*

DAVID R. HAMILTON PHD, AUTHOR OF *HOW YOUR MIND CAN HEAL YOUR BODY*

*'A healthy gut is not only the foundation of our physical health; it is also critical to our mental and emotional health. Equally, to heal our gut we can't just work with the physical aspects, we also have to work with our mind and emotions. Cara Wheatley-McGrain offers a practical and inspiring approach to gut healing on each of these levels, rooted in her own lived experience.'*

ALEX HOWARD, FOUNDER & CHAIRMAN OF THE OPTIMUM HEALTH CLINIC AND AUTHOR OF *DECODE YOUR FATIGUE*

*'Never before have I encountered a book on gut health that feels like a warm hug. In these sterile living conditions, knowledge of ways to boost our gut health is vital and* [Calm Your Gut] *manages to empower us with such heart and deep authenticity. Cara's lived experience cultivates a real sense of understanding, and I love the relatable and practical nature of her soothing suggestions. This is a welcome new approach to gut health, anchored in compassion, self-insight and real holistic health. So refreshing.'*

SUZY READING, PSYCHOLOGIST AND AUTHOR OF *SELF-CARE FOR TOUGH TIMES*

*'Cara has a wonderful style and brings what is perhaps our most underrated organ – the gut – to life. She has lovingly joined together personal experience, scientific research and expert advice, all embedded in compassion, to develop your must-have handbook for all things wellbeing.'*

DR JENNA MACCIOCHI, AUTHOR OF *IMMUNITY: THE SCIENCE OF STAYING WELL*

# CALM YOUR GUT

## A MINDFUL AND COMPASSIONATE GUIDE TO HEALING IBD AND IBS

CARA WHEATLEY-McGRAIN

HAY HOUSE
Carlsbad, California • New York City
London • Sydney • New Delhi

**Published in the United Kingdom by:**
Hay House UK Ltd, The Sixth Floor, Watson House,
54 Baker Street, London W1U 7BU
Tel: +44 (0)20 3927 7290; Fax: +44 (0)20 3927 7291; www.hayhouse.co.uk

**Published in the United States of America by:**
Hay House Inc., PO Box 5100, Carlsbad, CA 92018-5100
Tel: (1) 760 431 7695 or (800) 654 5126
Fax: (1) 760 431 6948 or (800) 650 5115; www.hayhouse.com

**Published in Australia by:**
Hay House Australia Pty Ltd, 18/36 Ralph St, Alexandria NSW 2015
Tel: (61) 2 9669 4299; Fax: (61) 2 9669 4144; www.hayhouse.com.au

**Published in India by:**
Hay House Publishers India, Muskaan Complex,
Plot No.3, B-2, Vasant Kunj, New Delhi 110 070
Tel: (91) 11 4176 1620; Fax: (91) 11 4176 1630; www.hayhouse.co.in



A catalogue record for this book is available from the British Library.

Tradepaper ISBN: 978-1-78817-814-3
E-book ISBN: 978-1-78817-582-1
Audiobook ISBN: 978-1-78817-610-1

Interior illustrations: p.xii, 6, 15, 30, 33, 34, 108: Jade Ho Design; all other illustrations: Kari Brownlie

FSC www.fsc.org MIX Paper from responsible sources FSC® C013056

Printed and bound in Great Britain by
TJ Books Limited, Padstow, Cornwall

*To my mum, Gerardine, you embody compassion in all you do.*

*To my husband, David, for your strength and kindness.*

*And to each and every gorgeous gut in the world – yes, I mean yours too!*

# CONTENTS


*About Calm Your Gut* xi

**Part I: Gut Knowledge** **1**

Chapter 1. How Your Gorgeous Gut Works 5

Chapter 2. Gut Self-knowledge 27

Chapter 3. Rewriting Your Gut Story 43

Chapter 4. Setting Healthy Gut Goals 51

**Part II: Gut Compassion** **59**

Chapter 5. The Anxious Gut 63

Chapter 6. The Compassionate Gut 75

Chapter 7. The Mindful Food Flow 83

Chapter 8. Sleep Care Is Gut Care 95

**Part III: Gut Healing** **111**

Chapter 9. Eliminate with Love 115

Chapter 10. The Resilient Gut 123

| | | |
|---|---|---|
| Chapter 11. | Healing the Fear in Flare | 145 |
| Chapter 12. | Movement and Microbiome | 165 |
| Chapter 13. | Gut Healing Dance | 173 |
| **Part IV: Gut Integrity** | | **183** |
| Chapter 14. | Becoming Gut Articulate | 187 |
| Chapter 15. | Your Gut Gang | 199 |
| Chapter 16. | The Sustainable Gut | 209 |
| **Part V: Gut-loving Food and Recipes** | | **221** |
| Chapter 17. | Fill Your Kitchen with Music and Gut-loving Soul | 225 |
| | Beautiful Brunches and Breakfasts | 229 |
| | Seasonal Smoothies | 235 |
| | Gut-soothing Soups | 237 |
| | Mindful Mains | 243 |
| | Desserts and Treats | 254 |
| *A Gorgeous Authentic Gut for Life* | | 259 |
| *Resources* | | 261 |
| *References* | | 267 |
| *Acknowledgements* | | 275 |
| *Index* | | 277 |
| *About the Author* | | 285 |

# ABOUT *CALM YOUR GUT*

Hey there. Don't skip this bit. I know you're tempted. That's you all over, rushing through to get to the main event. I want you to take a moment to understand the healing journey we are about to embark on. You won't need to acquire a whole new skill set or lots of facts. Oh yes, in Part I, there will be some new knowledge, but otherwise, it's more about taking stock, slowing right down and letting go of some stuff. To create a space to assimilate where you and your gut are right now and how to calm and heal.

I did my assimilating when my life veered off course in my twenties when I ended up in the hospital about to lose my colon. Well, that doesn't happen to everyone every day. Except it does happen to someone, somewhere every day.[1] I now know a lot about the gut and even more about the lifestyle changes to keep my dear gut calm and healthy.

I hope you're reading this because you care about your gut and want to sort it out. Although, to be honest, I'm not going to tell you how to *sort it out* or *fix it*. No, I'm going to tell you how to love it. How to love your gut so much that you learn to calm your gut naturally and organically. Those changes might happen slowly, but they will happen as sure as night turns to day. Because when you know just how to love and calm your unique gut – and I mean in a deep, gut-loving, wholesome way – it will change your life.

So, I wish you and your gut a big hug on the journey because, honestly, I've thought a lot about your gut. Yes, I really have. I thought about nothing else except your gut as I wrote this book: what it might need to know and what it might want to share with you.

## The gorgeous 4Gs to calm gut health

In creating calm gut health, we will explore the 4Gs: gut knowledge, gut compassion, gut healing and gut integrity. The 4Gs are not linear. Rather these four elements interweave to support you to live an authentic gut-led life.

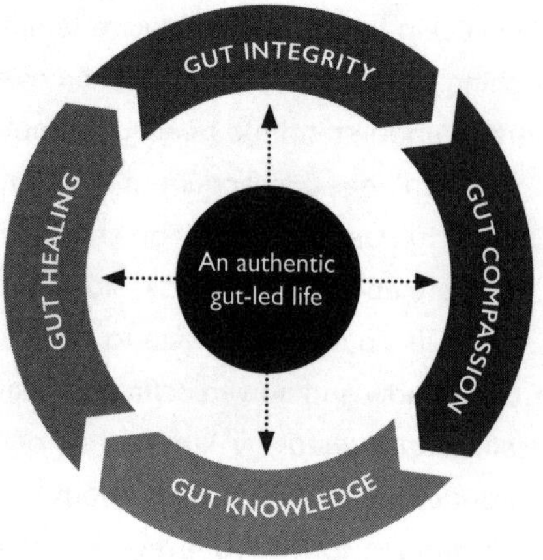


Figure 1: The 4Gs

**Part I: Gut Knowledge** shares the beautiful biology of your small and large intestine, so you can get to know your own gut and how it's doing right now. These are exciting times in the scientific understanding of the gut microbiome. We now know gut health is inextricably tied to the immune system and our susceptibility to disease. So, in a time when we want to stay well, getting to know our gorgeous gut has never been more important. The research is ongoing, so I encourage you to watch out for updates at carawheatleymcgrain.com to renew your own unique healing journey.

I'll also introduce you to the core practice of **base belly breathing**. This practice is a foundation training in mindful abdominal breathing to support your gut healing at both a physical and an energetic level. We'll spend a bit of time investigating the roots of your gut trouble, including a questionnaire to see how you're currently showing up for your gut, and we'll consider how you can reframe your gut story in a whole new way.

In **Part II**, we develop **Gut Compassion**. The practices here are designed to encourage you to complete an honest appraisal of your current stress points and where balance is missing in your life. We'll explore our sometimes-hidden gut-twisting emotions. I'll share the **mindful food flow principle**, which aims to reawaken your gut instincts through more mindful shopping. Throughout this section, we'll come back again to the mindful base belly breathing and deepen this practice with the addition of **Belly Metta Bhavana.** We'll also write a love letter from your gut.

**Part III** contains the practical steps to **Gut Healing** by being more mindful with your food and lifestyle choices. By this point, you'll have gained the confidence and motivation to follow the best advice available to construct your **personal elimination diet** – one of the keystones of good gut health. As Hippocrates said, 'Let food be thy medicine, and medicine be thy food.'

While recognizing that there are times when the only immediate solution is prescribed meds or even surgery, the scientific evidence is clear: diet impacts gut health. So, we will examine the radical impact of diet on your microbiome. I can attest personally, as can countless others, to the healing power of finding the right diet, physical movement and lifestyle choices to help heal your uniquely gorgeous gut. We will also discuss what we can do when things aren't going so well for our gut, and I'll share calming practices and affirmations to help you heal the fear in flare.

In **Part IV,** we'll continue to move towards physical and emotional **Gut Integrity**. Honouring your gut transforms illness into an opportunity to take stock and reflect deeply on your true purpose. We'll also explore what it means to be **health articulate** and how you can create a **gut gang** – a trusted network that will support you to maintain gut health and integrity. This includes preparing for medical appointments and strategies for difficult food situations. Alongside this, I want you to have fun with the **30 ways to love thy belly**. This practice aims to inspire you to be creative and playful in cultivating a loving relationship with your gut.

Finally, in **Part V: Gut-loving Food and Recipes**, I share a few of my everyday gut-healing recipes. We'll explore ways to naturally diversify your personal food map and build up confidence in using the secret gut-loving power of the 3Ps: probiotics, prebiotics and polyphenols.

## My gut story

I've been tracking the latest gut health developments because I am deeply invested in what it means: I'm living with *incurable* IBD (inflammatory bowel disease). IBD is a chronic health condition that causes sections of the bowel to become inflamed and painful. I have pan ulcerative colitis (the whole of my large intestine has been affected by inflammation) and suffer from IBS (irritable bowel syndrome). This functional gut disorder leads to bloating and discomfort.

I've been successfully managing the conditions with as few traditional prescription drugs as possible and finding alternative healing approaches. Over the last two decades, I've been fortunate to have long spells of deep remission and rare early-stage symptoms, which I have managed to heal. As I do this, I continue to ask challenging questions:

- How do we make sense of the science to commit to the right actions to heal our gorgeous gut?
- How can we understand our illness to heal ourselves, not just of the symptoms of IBD and IBS, but also of the underlying causes?

And the million-dollar question:

- How do we make sustained positive changes in our life?

I'll leave those questions there for now, but we'll come back to them. For now, I'd like to share my gut health story.

In spring 2001, I was at university, having recently been diagnosed with IBD. I'd been fine, almost like the whole thing (the diagnosis) was a mistake, a one-off. But despite trying to convince myself that I wasn't sick, I had become too weak to walk, hadn't been able to eat a proper meal in months, had a gnawing pain in my gut, and spent so many hours on the toilet I had set up camp in the family bathroom. Little did I know the disease had sparked a fire in my system, and it was getting worse, and the day my lovely mum drove me to the hospital is distilled into distinct slices of memory.

The serious face of the A&E registrar who set up my drip. The shock of seeing the dark globules of blood pouring out of me. The moment the gastric consultant took my mum to one side and told her I had 48 hours to respond to the intravenous steroids before they would need to operate to remove the overheated twist of flesh – the remnants of my colon.

That night on the dark ward, I wake to see shifting pinpoints of light and the voices of two women nearby. I experience a strange sensation. I am no longer in my body but at a distance, stretched out and shapeless. An intravenous drip seeps its steady stream of steroids into my blood, waves of a deep tiredness wash over me. I try to tune in to the women's voices, 'Her blood pressure's still way too low. She'll need another drip.' I fall into darkness.

The next day I wake up to my exhausted body. I feel overwhelming compassion, like looking through the wrong end of a telescope. Like I have stepped away from myself and can see this other me.

Weeks of hospital recovery are followed by slow months of rehabilitation as I'm weaned off intravenous steroids. Back home, I start the real healing as I begin to learn about the forgotten inner world of my gut. And, well, my colon and I are here to tell the tale – I was one of the lucky ones. The moral of this story? Sometimes to survive, you have to take some heavy-ass drugs. Each of our gut stories is unique to us. But I say with my hand on my heart and my gut: the key to **thriving** with IBD or IBS is vastly different.

*My gut tells me compassion is the key.*

When I started my journey, there were no studies to back up my idea that radical self-care can calm and heal the gut, just a deep instinct that I needed to make profound changes to how I was showing up for my gut. What's exciting now is that science has caught up, and recent studies show that **self-compassion can reduce inflammation in the body.**[2]

What I hope you take from this book is that your gut is made up of some tremendous organs that daily transform the food you eat into energy for life. They do this tirelessly, quietly, in the background of our lives, but every now and then, you get a message from your gut's deep, dark recesses that things are not quite right. So, if you're suffering from IBD, one of the best things you can do is get curious. Really curious. When you get compassionately curious, you might start to ask: Why do some folk get sick, and some don't? Why do we sometimes get so seriously ill with IBD, and other times we manage to step back from the brink?

This book will help you tune in to your unique gut story and answer these questions. My aspiration would be for you to learn to love, cherish and calm your gorgeous gut.

So, take a deep breath. Yes, don't skip past that part either.

Take a deep breath, and let's begin.

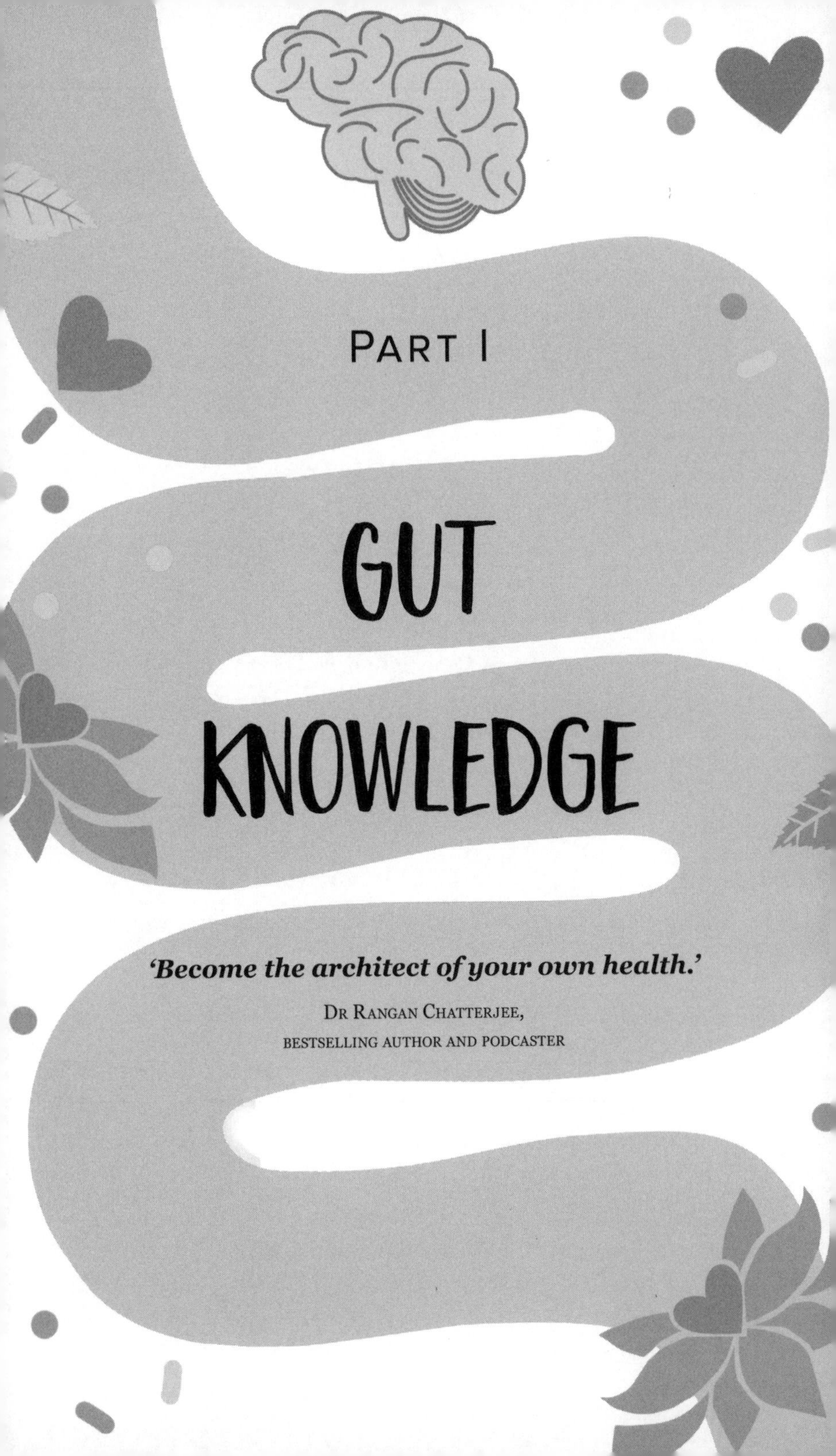

## Part I

# GUT KNOWLEDGE

***'Become the architect of your own health.'***

Dr Rangan Chatterjee,
bestselling author and podcaster

Information is power when it comes to calming your gut. If you're here because you're tired of your endless hard bloated belly, I see you. If you're reading this because you've tried everything and feel like you're going one step forwards, two steps back, in an endless cycle of flare and remission, I'm with you. If you think that others don't quite get how hard it is living with a troubled gut, I know you. It can feel like lonely work this healing. But I would say to you and your dear gut, you've got this. It's time to begin to breathe deeply into that beautiful belly of yours.

If your gut is troubled, you're not alone. Every 30 minutes, someone in the UK is diagnosed with IBD; that's nearly half a million people. There are over three million inflamed intestines in the USA and Canada, while Australians have one of the highest IBD incidences per capita. Bloated, inflamed and too often unloved and unheeded, 10 million tummies in the UK regularly suffer from IBS. Many sufferers don't even make it to their GP, choosing to muddle through their gut trouble solo. The vast majority of those with a troubled gut live in the West. Scientists have also noticed a new trend: gut trouble is spreading into new territories. Places and people with no previous history of gut health diseases.[1] Has gut health reached a crisis point, and why?

Gut knowledge is the fertile soil in which gut compassion and gut healing grow. As you get to know your tender gut, that velvety jejunum and wondrous colon, you'll see them as the loveable unsung heroes and heroines of your life. We'll start by exploring the digestive tract system and how it works, then dive into inflammation – what it is and how even early life events can have a long-term impact on the health of your gut bacteria. You'll learn about the intricate biology of your very own uniquely gorgeous gut through a series of exercises and guided visualizations. We'll also start to unravel your personal gut narrative, so you're ready to rewrite the next chapter and set your gut-life goals.

This new gut knowledge reveals just how important it is to take care of this precious piece of inner kit. So, come explore with curiosity, and an open mind and heart.

## CHAPTER 1

# HOW YOUR GORGEOUS GUT WORKS

*'The human body has a ringmaster. This ringmaster controls your digestion, your immunity, your brain, your weight, your health and even your happiness. This ringmaster is the gut.'*

NANCY S. MURE, AUTHOR OF *EAT! – EMPOWER. ADJUST. TRIUMPH!*

I believe there is a path to calming our troubled gut. We've just got to take the time to put our own healing jigsaw together piece by little piece. Let's start right at the beginning with the digestive tract and gut biology, and after that, we'll move on to the good gut-loving stuff. And, well, that's the secret. You've got to learn to love your gut.

Gut health is a hot topic right now. Mainly because of an exciting new area of research that's emerging front and centre of the gut health debate. You've probably heard about it: the **gut microbiome**. But let's start by taking a closer look at our gorgeous gut; and when I say gut, I'm referring to the whole of the digestive system from input to output.

## How the digestive system works

Digestion begins in the mouth, with the physical process of breaking down food with your teeth and digestive juices being released into the saliva. So right now, think about your favourite food. What happens? Yep, you get that mouth-watering sensation. The sight, smell, even thinking about food triggers your body to get ready to digest. You've probably heard the expression 'we eat with our eyes first' and, well, there's a lot to be said for that, but as you'll see, that's just the start of the process.

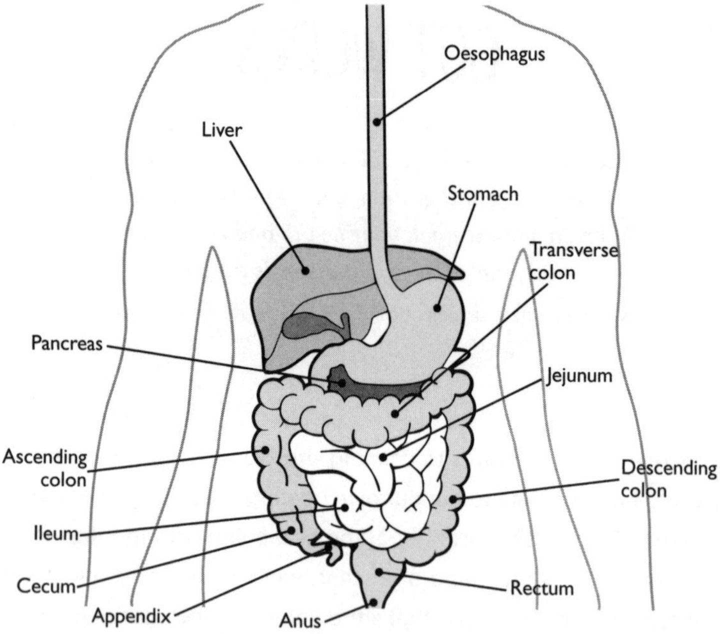


Figure 2: The digestive system

One of the key enzymes released by the salivary glands is amylase, which helps break down starchy foods, such as bread and potatoes. As you chew, food is broken down into smaller particles. The stomach doesn't have teeth, so thoroughly chewing your food can support the digestive process's latter stages.

Once you swallow, your food starts its journey through the 9m (29ft 6in) digestive tract. First, the munched-up particles head down the 25cm (10in) oesophagus into your stomach. If you've ever eaten on the run, this is where some of your tasty meal can get stuck, creating that nub in your throat or upper chest. Hello, too, to acid reflux. This happens when the sphincter between the oesophagus and stomach is weakened. To support the onward momentum of food, there are a series of sphincters (which act a bit like airtight seals) along the digestive tract. Food moves in a one-way motion in a series of peristaltic waves, triggered when you eat.

The stomach is positioned in the upper left of the abdomen in a large, stretchy, J-shaped pouch that can expand to hold your Friday night takeout or contract overnight when it's empty. Your stomach, lined with a thick layer of protective mucus, continues the chemical and physical digestion process in its strongly acidic environment with a pH of 1.5–3.5. You know when you have missed your lunch, and you hear that tummy gurgle? Well, this is a sign that your body thinks it's time to eat. The body produces an astounding 2L (3½pt) of gastric juices each day.

Your food usually spends two to five hours in the stomach, turning slowly into a liquid called chyme, which is released in short bursts through the pyloric sphincter into the duodenum, the first section of your small intestine (*see figure 5, page 33*). This liquid then continues to move through the next two sections of the small intestine: the jejunum and ileum. The small intestine is a fascinating piece of kit. It's long and narrow, and if you unfurled it right out, it would form a long sausage-like tube stretching across the room for 6m (19ft 8in). Pretty extraordinary, hey?

The small intestine is an intricately layered system for extracting as many nutrients as possible from your food. The surface is covered in a layer of 1mm (0.04in) finger-like villi, and if you look closer still, these tiny villi are covered in a further layer of microvilli, interwoven with blood vessels. This ingenious design increases the intestine's surface area to a whopping 250m$^2$ (2,700ft$^2$) – that's around the size of a tennis court. It's here in the small intestine that 90 per cent of food absorption and digestion occurs.

The muscles lining the small intestine help mix food with digestive juices from the pancreas and liver. These enzymes help break down carbohydrates, fats and proteins, while the small intestine walls absorb water and the digested nutrients into your bloodstream. Food usually takes between two and six hours to travel through the small intestine. As it does, it triggers peristaltic waves, which start to move the waste products of the digestive process into the large intestine.

The large intestine (also known as the colon) is shorter at around 1–1.5m (3ft 3in–4ft 11in) and fatter, with three key sections: the ascending, transverse and descending colon. As you can see from figure 2 on page 6, the large intestine looks a bit like a three-sided picture frame around the small intestine, wrapped up and layered inside the abdominal cavity. Right at the centre of this intricate art installation is your magical microbiome, containing billions of bacteria that are as unique to each of us as our fingerprints. This diverse mix of bacteria contains around 70 per cent of your immune system, and the colon also supports the synthesis of vitamins B and K.

This final part of your digestive process is also the slowest. Eliminating the waste products from your food can vary between a rapid 10 and a sluggish 59 hours. During this time, your colon absorbs water and creates poop. Sluggish colons tend towards constipation; too fast, and you have the opposite – diarrhoea.

In total, the transit time from food input (evening meal) to poop output is between 10 hours (next morning) or a much longer 73 hours (three days later). Take home message:

*What you eat can stick around*
*for quite a while.*

## Gut microbiome

The gut biome is used to describe the bacteria populating the gut and is sometimes called the 'second genome'. So how many bugs do you have? Well, the 4,000 species have a population of around 100 trillion, which are right now nestled in the intricate folds of your large intestine. Wow. We have co-evolved with this fantastic array of tiny beings. It turns out we simply can't live a happy, healthy life without them.

While scientists are busily trying to map the genome, what's becoming clear is that there's a relationship between the increase in gut problems and the typical Western microbiome. And because the diversity and complexity of the bacteria that live on and in us are far greater than our own human DNA, we cannot just draw simple conclusions from this complex conundrum. But there's pretty compelling evidence that those of us with gut health issues have a reduced range of gut bacteria, and those of us with IBD and IBS appear to have an imbalance in the profile of our gut bugs compared with healthy people.[2]

We'll talk more about the weird and wonderful world of your microbiome and how it impacts your broader wellbeing throughout *Calm Your Gut*.[3] For now, it's worth reminding yourself that with this level of complexity, there are so many ways that the gut can struggle. IBS is one of the most common gut diagnoses in the West, but there are other conditions like diverticulitis, small intestine bacterial overgrowth (SIBO), gastritis, IBD and many more. We're going to take a closer look at IBS and IBD, but the strategies shared apply to a wide array of gut health issues.

So, let's turn the spotlight on one of the most common ways our guts can trouble us – IBS.

## The essential guide to IBS

A whopping one in five of us will suffer some IBS symptoms, and around one in 10 will experience deeply distressing, life-restricting symptoms. IBS is frequently described as a functional condition, meaning that there is limited evidence of physiological changes to the gut wall. For many years, the lack of evidence of physical changes meant people suffering debilitating symptoms were told, 'It's all in your head.'

Fortunately, the world has moved on, and medical practitioners recognize that IBS unquestionably impacts life quality. Symptoms include bloating, discomfort, pain, diarrhoea, constipation, cramping and nausea, amongst others. As with any gut imbalance, diagnosis takes time and often involves some pretty invasive tests. While this book can help you heal your gut, you should always visit your doctor and ask for a formal diagnosis for any bloating or digestive issues. Although more rarely, these symptoms can indicate other more serious conditions, including some cancers, so always avoid self-diagnosis.

Gut health distress can also cause a significant amount of time off work. Whilst the condition is now widely known, and many of us have direct experience of it, it's still common to avoid sharing this with managers at work,[4] increasing the sense of isolation and anxiety.

Curiously, IBS has become a kind of 'catch all' term for what may prove to be a more complex array of underlying gut health issues that we are only just starting to fully unravel. It turns out a lot can go wrong with our guts. I'm sure everyone knows something about the bloating, unbuttoning unease of indigestion. But there's a more serious side to this occasional discomfort because we're discovering that gut health has wide-ranging implications for our health, including our immune system. So, let's turn the spotlight on a more serious gut disease: IBD.

## IBD

There are two primary forms of IBD: ulcerative colitis (UC) and Crohn's disease (CD). Inflammation is the root of most diseases, for example, arthritis, laryngitis, gastritis. *Itis* comes from Greek, meaning 'inflammation'. In Crohn's disease, the *itis* doesn't obey particular rules; it can affect any part of the intestinal system. In ulcerative colitis, the *itis* is limited to the large intestine. The colon becomes sore and inflamed, which can lead to ulcers and bleeding. The main symptoms are diarrhoea, pain, fever and weight loss. It's quite common to have remission periods interspersed with more severe flares, which may delay initial diagnosis.

In Crohn's disease, inflammation occurs across different sections of the small and large intestine, with places of more serious damage to the intestinal wall layers, which can thicken and become inflamed. As with ulcerative colitis, gut inflammation causes widespread problems throughout the body. It's pretty common in Crohn's disease to experience other autoimmune issues, including arthritis, skin conditions, and inflammation of the eyes and mouth. What's less well known is that people living with ulcerative colitis and Crohn's disease may experience fatigue, exhaustion and nutritional deficiencies, and have a higher risk of bowel cancer.

The most common first-line treatments for IBD are NSAIDs (non-steroidal anti-inflammatory drugs). More persistent flares are treated with steroids or biologics, which inhibit inflammation by targeting and suppressing the body's immune-system response. However, these life-saving meds can have a range of unwanted side effects, including reduced immune function and longer-term increased risk of osteoporosis.

The likelihood of requiring surgery in Crohn's disease is pretty high. It's less common in ulcerative colitis, but still impacts around one in five people. The good news is early diagnosis, and better treatment regimens mean rates of surgery are reducing. But IBD remains a pain in the proverbial ass – quite literally. I know for some, an ostomy (stoma to replace part of the bowel) is a positive choice – a courageous decision after a long, wearying battle. To each of you, I salute your courage, whatever your story. I love the brave folk on Instagram who share their ostomy photos in their bikinis and boxers. Go, brave ones. If there's ever been a time to connect and share, it's right now.

As I said earlier, what's important to know as you read this, is that if you have an unhappy gut, you're not alone. When I walk down the high street, I can see many opportunities to eat the stuff that will damage my guts. It's all-pervasive, easily accessible and cheap. But what else happens in a city that has such an impact on our wellbeing? Thich Nhat Hanh writes of the city as a place we experience:

> *... pressure of time, noise and pollution, the lonely crowds – these have all been created by the disruptive course of our economic growth. They are all sources of mental illness (and stress).*[5]

Over the coming chapters, we'll explore stress points in our lives and techniques to counteract anxiety and look at how this may play an essential role in supporting our gut health. For now, we've looked at some of the BIG data, and we'll come back to this big picture again and again on our mindful gut journey, but I want to stay firmly focused on you – the person newly diagnosed or long-term living with IBD or IBS.

## Understanding inflammation

Inflammation is a healthy response, a reaction of your body trying to heal and re-establish balance. When inflammation arises in any part of your gut, you will almost certainly experience pain, particularly after eating. The whole process of food moving through the digestive tract will cause anything from mild discomfort to full-on agony. Imagine rubbing food against a skin abrasion. In your gut, the tiny raw villi and delicate parts of the sensitized ileum are invisible to us but interwoven with our enteric nervous system, containing 100 million neurons.

It turns out our guts are sensitive. In fact, it is sometimes called the second brain. The gut communicates to the brain all the time through the vagus nerve, and it's this nerve that may well explain the power of our gut instinct. *Vagus* comes from the Latin 'to wander', as the vagus nerve traces a path from the brain along the right side of the neck into the chest, through to the gut. It's this nerve that may well explain the power of our gut instinct. The vagus nerve plays a crucial part in shaping the inflammatory responses in the gut. Micro levels of inflammation and sensitivity, causing changes to the intestinal wall, may be triggered by many things, including the foods we eat.

There are two main types of allergic responses triggered by the foods we eat: immunoglobulin E response (IgE) and immunoglobulin G response (IgG).

## *Immunoglobulin E response (IgE)*

A rapid response allergy, an IgE mediated response, is a powerful autoimmune reaction, and potentially anaphylaxis. The most common of these are due to nut allergies. There have been some tragic, high-profile cases that have led to increased awareness and, in the UK, a requirement by law for more transparent labelling of food. **Natasha's Law** was pioneered by Natasha Ednan-Laperouse's parents after their daughter died from an allergic reaction to sesame seeds from a café-bought baguette in 2016.[6]

There's been an explosion in the number of us experiencing food allergies in recent years. This may in part be explained by our more sterile living conditions. This theory forms part of a more complex picture of how our immune system can overreact to small triggers in dramatic ways – think pollen allergy, for example.

### *Immunoglobulin G response (IgG)*

The more common and widespread IgG response is less severe, indicating a milder intolerance to foods. This delayed response includes irritation, bloating and discomfort. Some of the most common allergens are dairy, gluten and corn. It is possible to remove some common food allergens for a short period as part of an elimination diet. We'll take a closer look at this in Part III: Gut Healing.

In IBD, the *itis* is not merely **on** or **off**; there's a scale of inflammation caused by many different triggers. When we experience inflammation, there is a powerful biochemical response. The body builds higher levels of C-reactive protein, a key inflammatory marker. Inflammation can also lead to a cycle of over-sensitized gut tissue and a leaky gut. The most accurate measure of gut inflammation is faecal calprotectin (which measures the presence of inflammatory markers in your poop).

## What even is a leaky gut?

You could be forgiven for being a little confused because there's been some dispute about this phrase. A leaky gut is all about **intestinal permeability.** Leading proponents of this theory, such as Zach Busch MD,[7] suggest that as the tight junctures of the cells in the gut wall become inflamed and swollen, this permeability leads to low-level chronic inflammation. The potential triggers that damage our delicate gut wall are manifold: highly processed foods, environmental pollutants, genetically modified (GM) foods, trace elements of fertilizers in our water and diet.[8] In a nutshell, Western living.

Once this chronic low-level inflammation occurs, the gut wall is less effective in filtering out large macromolecules (endotoxins), which leak into the bloodstream. The immune cells try to attack foreign invaders by producing further inflammatory compounds. This can create a cycle of chronic systemic inflammation in the gut and body.

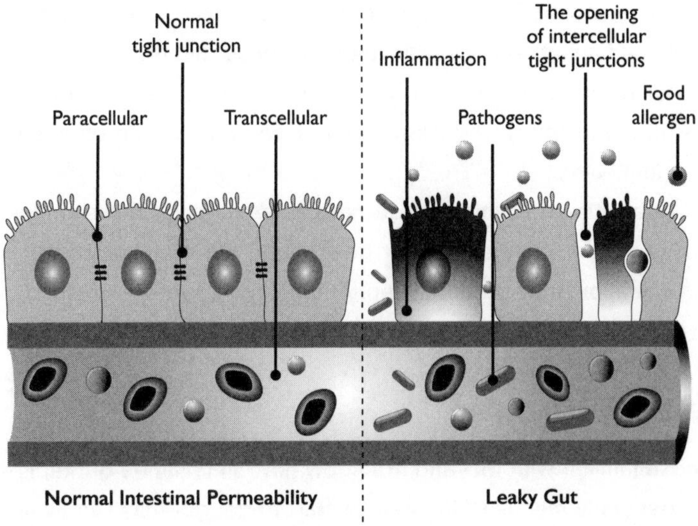


Figure 3: The gut wall and the cycle of chronic inflammation

There's evidence that increased intestinal permeability may contribute to gut health issues like IBD and IBS,[9] but unravelling cause and effect is tricky. IBD may cause damage to the epithelial layer of the gut and the tight junctures of the gut lining. Still, there's also evidence that gastritis (stomach inflammation, triggered by diet, excessive alcohol, medications or Helicobacter pylori infection) can have a long-term impact on the health of the gut lining. Intestinal permeability may also play a role in a much broader spectrum of autoimmune diseases, including arthritis, Alzheimer's disease, allergies, acne, type 2 diabetes and obesity.

It's important to share that some traditional mainstream medical thinking doesn't support the theory of intestinal permeability as a factor in gut health and autoimmune conditions.[10] But the picture is evolving, and a damaged, permeable gut is currently accepted as playing a role in the interplay between gut health and wellbeing.

There has been a rapid rise in recent decades in our exposure to chemicals and pollutants both in our food and environment. There are other factors involved, of course, but it makes sense that this could be impacting the sensitive organs of our gut and the balance of our ancient, co-evolving microbiome. In fact, even short-term disruption of the gut's microbes can have long-lasting effects on our gut health.[11]

A sensitized and inflamed gut can cause bloating and discomfort. These subtle changes in your health, and the early indicators of inflammation, may go unnoticed. At times when you're stressed or overworked, subtle early warning signs simply get lost.

## Gut-fully self-aware

Those familiar with IBD and IBS know how an inflamed gut feels – *itis* generally means PAIN. As you start to get gut-fully self-aware, you may notice how stress triggers your gut health. To explore the role of stress, you need to understand how your gut and brain work together across the gut–brain axis, recognizing the vagus nerve as a key player in your gut–brain alliance.

### *The stressed-out gut*

Have you ever noticed how your appetite is impacted by how you feel? When you are anxious, depressed or stressed, you may overeat or struggle to eat at all. Either way, your digestive system will be off-kilter. A little short-term stress is OK, but when we experience stress in a sustained way, it becomes a problem and impacts the gut in some specific ways.

Your gut and brain are connected by the vagus nerve. Its job is to communicate information straight from your organs (specifically the gut) to the brain, and it's a bi-directional relationship. If you've never heard of it, it's about time you had an introduction.

This long, wandering nerve starts at the base of your brain below the ears, along the side of the throat, the heart and lungs and into the gut. And this is why it's so fascinating. The vagus nerve is woven into the wall of the intestine. So, what happens in the vagus never just stays in the vagus. It turns out that the vagus plays a key role in supporting our physical and mental health.[12]

What does that *mean* for you and your gut?

As humans, we live between two key states: with our sympathetic or our parasympathetic nervous system activated. When we are stressed, the brain triggers the adrenal glands to release the hormones adrenaline and cortisol. These hormones feed a series of responses. Under stress, our (un) sympathetic nervous system is dominant. Okay, I've added the 'un' as I always find the 'sympathetic' nervous system label unhelpful. When we are in stress mode, we are in our flight-or-fight readiness.

In flight or fight, our bodies divert blood to the muscles and heart ready to flee or fight, and this reduces the blood supply to the gut. Sometimes we may even experience an overwhelming need to lose our load (pee or poop ourselves). Whilst all this is happening, digestive juices get repressed. We don't need a hamburger and a side order of fries when we're getting ready for flight or fight. So less saliva, fewer gastric juices.

Imagine your ancestors out hunting a big, scary animal. Yikes. The stress response was a super-efficient and sensible system. It worked well for that kind of sudden, high-risk situation. Big, frightening animal: cortisol floods our system, increasing fat and sugar levels in the bloodstream to feed our muscles ready for action. That's why, after a bout of stress, you may feel depleted (sound familiar)? Right after a stressful event, you have a strong biological pull to refuel and thousands of years of evolution mean you're more likely to head for high-fat, easy-sugar energy. That cocktail of surging stress hormones acts to shut down digestion (constipation) or speed it up (diarrhoea). Take home message: when we eat in stress mode (rushed lunches, rapid-fire dinners), our gut struggles.

## *Back to the vagus*

The vagus nerve aligns with your parasympathetic nervous system – the rest, reset and digest system. This is the state in which you want to spend more time. Especially when you're eating. The vagus nerve activation means blood supply returns from the muscles and heart back to the inner organs, ready for digestion, the salivary glands start flowing, heart rate decreases and breathing naturally slows. YEAH, so good.

We can acknowledge just how much we're easy prey to adrenaline – a gut wash of cortisol. Too much traffic, an interview, a row, and our heart rate goes up. Thanks to Fitbit and co, these days, we can actually see this in action. In these moments, our gut closes down. When we get *really* clear gut-led knowledge on just how much eating on the go and general levels of stress impact the gut, we can set out to make changes. So as part of the process of learning to take *gut care* of yourself, we'll explore some practical ways of taking a calm approach to eating in Parts II and III.

## *Why is stress so bad for your gorgeous gut?*

We've covered the effect of adrenaline on the gut. Let's step out and look at the BIG picture again. Right now, most of us are living a standard Western lifestyle, the kind of 24-7 world our ancient biome has never had to navigate before.

My most severe IBD episode followed studying in a crowded flat in London and dealing with a broken heart. Cue stress overload, anxious *itis* in my gut and, well, you know how the story goes. Over half of patients who have an IBD flare say it was triggered by stressful life events.[6] Let's face it, living in a modern city can be fun and frazzling, and stress triggers can be cumulative rather than isolated. As Thomas Merton said: 'The rush and pressure of modern life are a form, perhaps the most modern-day form of its innate violence.'[13] Sometimes we can feel stretched thin across the competing demands of our lives, saturated by the sheer amount of stuff that fills our days. So time to make space for some gut reflection.

## Gut-loving Journal

Journalling is a great place to record your personal gut knowledge and create space to deepen your understanding of your triggers. So, take a breath. It's time to start your very own Gut-loving Journal.

As you continue through the exercises in this book, things will come up for you. This journal is the place you bear witness and track your changes. Journalling is a neat way of self-coaching. It expedites your learning.

Take a few minutes to reflect on a recent gut flare that you've experienced. What were your triggers? Work, uncertainty, relationships? Just take a moment to reflect on what you and your guts have been through. Be honest. But don't be too tough on yourself. We're each unique and can experience the same circumstance differently.

The truth is 'tough love' – you know the kind (the white-knuckle, holding-on-for-dear-life and having-stern-words-with-yourself) yeah, that kind – doesn't actually calm your gut. Not in a way that is long-term and sustainable. We're going to look at how to stop the tough love in more detail in Part II: Gut Compassion, and the anxious gut and why being tough is not a winning combination. But right now, take a moment to reflect on your starting point. The following questionnaire is designed to get you thinking about where you are right now.

## Get-to-know-your-gut questionnaire

I know from personal experience that having a gut that doesn't work well can be frustrating. It can feel like *hard work* and, of course, darn painful. In the midst of this, we can feel disconnected and confused. So how are you getting on with your gut?

1. **Which foods or diet feels right for you?**

   ● You have tried out a range of different diets and started to identify the foods that have an impact on your gut wellbeing and general health.

   ■ You're not sure about all these different diets. Some of it feels like 'spin'. You trust your doctor and NHS dietician.

   ★ You have been trying lots of different approaches. You may have tried gluten-free/dairy-free/low FODMAP. For a short time, they appear to work, but after a while, you feel bloated and unwell again.

   ▲ You are confused about how what you eat impacts your gut.

2. **How do you feel about alternative approaches to treating your gut health condition?**

   ● You are open to engaging with alternative health approaches like acupuncture, functional medicine, etc.

   ■ You stick with and trust the medicines that your doctor prescribes.

   ★ You've been meaning to get some nutritional advice but haven't had time to follow through.

   ▲ You follow online forums and chat with others that share your condition.

3. **Do you find there's a relationship between stress and your gut?**
   - ● You have a sense that your gut health problems are linked to stress and high-anxiety situations.
   - ■ You've had gut health issues for as long as you can remember. It's just how it is for you.
   - ★ You've practised yoga and mindfulness, and you notice that these seem to ease some of your worst symptoms, but sometimes nothing works.
   - ▲ There seems to be no pattern to your flares. You can't understand what triggers are impacting your gut.

4. **How do you feel when talking with other people about your gut health?**
   - ● You find it natural to connect with your own feelings and can express them to others.
   - ■ You get uncomfortable at the idea of opening up. It's not the thing you do in your family.
   - ★ You're usually happy to journal, and it helps you process your thoughts so you don't burden others.
   - ▲ You are generally OK to talk about it, but you're careful who you speak to.

5. **If you have a flare, you...**
   - ● Always try to make time for a bit of self-pampering.
   - ■ Knuckle down with your regime and hope it will pass, and you'll get over it. You think the term 'self-care' is fluffy. You need to be tough on yourself. That's the only way to get results.
   - ★ Read a book or take some inspiration from social media.
   - ▲ Try to take some time out, but it depends on what is happening. Sometimes the demands of life mean it's not possible.

6. **Do you find there's a relationship between your lifestyle and your gut?**
   - ● You can generally make changes and improve your life and health for the better.
   - ■ Life just happens. Flare-ups and bloating happen. You just have to deal with it and get on.
   - ★ Sometimes it's tough. But you're on the journey to change and try to take each day at a time.
   - ▲ You're unsure about where to begin with the lifestyle changes you think you need to make.

7. **If you had to choose your least helpful character trait, it would be...**
   - ● Lack of self-compassion.
   - ■ Impatience.
   - ★ Worry or anxiety.
   - ▲ Overthinking.

8. **You always feel better when you...**
   - ● Breathe deeply and spend time in nature.
   - ■ Get things off your chest.
   - ★ Share your feelings in a journal or with others.
   - ▲ Just take some time to yourself and have a break from technology or social media.

9. **When things don't work out, you're most likely to think...**
   - ● Things always have a purpose.
   - ■ Life's not fair.
   - ★ Just your luck.
   - ▲ Things have a way of working out.

10. **In terms of your current gut health plan (if you have a current diagnosis), you feel like...**
    - ● You understand each of the meds that you have been prescribed, including the benefits and side effects.
    - ■ You trust your doctor to prescribe the right thing for you. You don't like to ask questions; you just want to focus on getting results.
    - ★ You hate the idea of being on meds for the rest of your life.
    - ▲ You have a good overall knowledge of your meds regime. You've tried a few and keep hoping the right one will work for you.

11. **At breakfast and lunch, you tend to...**
    - ● Always try to appreciate the food, especially if you've spent time creating it.
    - ■ Just eat. It really doesn't make a difference how you eat. You get bloated whatever you do.
    - ★ Always intend to eat slowly and try to appreciate it, but forget and find yourself having seconds before you notice.
    - ▲ It varies on the time of day and what's happening. You get distracted and sometimes blink, and the food is gone.

12. **At evening mealtimes, you tend to...**
    - ● Spend time being present with your plate of food and share what's happening.
    - ■ Finish up a work project, eating what's left on your plate one-handed.
    - ★ Reach for the remote and flick between your favourite TV shows.
    - ▲ Try your best to be aware of what you're eating but usually forget.

13. **After a meal you...**

- ● Feel satiated and give yourself some time to simply digest.
- ■ Barely notice as you've been eating while multi-tasking, checking your emails, watching TV, etc.
- ★ Feel like you should sit still for a little while because you know it's the right thing to do but end up doing tasks for others.
- ▲ You remember some of the time to allow yourself to digest, but under pressure or when distracted, you forget.

14. **When do you experience bloating?**

- ● I notice bloating after eating specific foods or a really large meal.
- ■ I feel bloated **all** the time.
- ★ Most of the time, whatever I eat.
- ▲ Occasionally. I'm still trying to work out the cause.

15. **When you're away from home and low on energy, you're most likely to reach for...**

- ● Some healthy homemade treats that you packed.
- ■ Whatever is to hand.
- ★ Sweets or a sugary drink because a treat occasionally is fine.
- ▲ A handful of nuts/seeds.

16. **How much do you feel you know about your gut biology?**

- ● You feel you know your body and your biology well.
- ■ You know enough, it's the doctor's job to diagnose and fix the situation.
- ★ You know there are quite a few different parts of the digestive system but don't always feel confident in naming them when

you are with a medical practitioner. Sometimes you feel overwhelmed by the technical terms when you try and speak to your doctor/consultant.

▲ You can label all the sections of your large and small intestine. If you're ever unsure, you research.

17. **How much do you share about your gut health issues with others?**
    - ● I have a trusted group of people I can chat to when I am flaring.
    - ■ I tend to deal with my flare on my own.
    - ★ I don't like to overshare, but I do follow others on social media and I find it comforting to know I'm not alone.
    - ▲ Sometimes I just need to talk, and I seek out people who understand how I feel.

18. **How much is your diet shaped by gut-led foods or intuitive eating?**
    - ● You integrate a diverse and varied diet to maintain your microbiome.
    - ■ You tend to eat what you like, and there are some foods in your diet that you cannot live without.
    - ★ You are pretty clear on what you want to reduce, but sometimes other life pressures make it hard to follow through.
    - ▲ You have a sense of the best foods, but sometimes there are so many mixed messages you get confused.

## How are you getting on with your gut?

**Mostly ● answers** – You have a good overall awareness of your gut health, and you are pretty clear on how your diet impacts your gut. You seek out alternative medicines at times. To deepen your gut health, you are keen to learn more and be consistent in your gut care. Take time looking at gut integrity and explore the recipes in Part V.

**Mostly ■ answers** – You're sometimes frustrated with your body. You feel it lets you down. Your frustration means you don't invest the time you need to ensure healing occurs across your body, mind and gut. It's time to invest in self-care. Spend time developing your gut knowledge and compassion so that you can start to build good gut health. Use journalling and start connecting with a broader gut gang that will support you.

**Mostly ★ answers** – You are confident in your gut biology, but you don't always put yourself and your gut first! You have lapses in your wellbeing because although you have a good sense of what you feel you *should* be doing, you don't always invest the time you need to actually do it, as sometimes you are too busy putting others' needs above your own. You're in the right place to start to explore your deeper feelings and how to build new compassionate rituals of self-care and establish a better support with your wider gut gang, which we'll explore in Part IV.

**Mostly ▲ answers** – At times, you feel a little confused about your gut and what's the right thing to do. You do some great things some of the time, but you're inconsistent, which means your gut isn't happy and you're unclear on how your actions and your health all link up. Your diet, lifestyle and gut are not fully aligned yet, leading to a range of gut health and broader wellbeing problems. You're in the right place to start your gut health journey. Take time to look at the practical exercises across Parts II and III to help you establish greater gut compassion and healing

---

Wow. Now you've got more information to work with, let's dive into gut self-knowledge.

## CHAPTER 2

# GUT SELF-KNOWLEDGE

*'What you seek is also seeking you.'*

RUMI, SUFI POET

How's your gut doing today?

There's a tendency to treat the digestive tract as a bit of a garbage disposal chute. Chuck a lot of stuff down there, usually mindlessly and way too fast. Then poke it with a large broom handle when things inevitably get stuck – perhaps some antacids for bloat or ibuprofen for discomfort.

If you're living with IBD and IBS, this whole scenario gets way more complex. By the time you end up in a doctor's surgery or hospital, it's like taking your car to your local garage. We want someone to look under the bonnet and fix it up, so we can jump right back in and drive. With the body, there is a real temptation to fixate on getting a *label*. Once we get the right diagnosis, that neat little label, our expectation is we will jump right back behind the wheel of our lives.

Conventional medical approaches are shaped by data. Patterns, big numbers and the idea of an abstract 'typical patient'. All well and good. Without mainstream medicine, I would have lost my lovely colon. But there's a hidden part to this, the idea of the 'hero doctor'. You know the person in a white coat who sorts all your shit out – quite literally in the case of gut trouble! The doctor orders tests, writes on a pad, looks reassuring, in control, and you go along with their advice. But there's another version – a vision of feeling more empowered about your body and your gut.

For example, 20 years ago, following an allergy test at my local health-food store, I stopped eating wheat. I saw an immediate improvement in my symptoms – lighter, less *itis*. When I shared this with my gastroenterologist, he blinked and said, 'There's no clinical evidence, unless you have coeliac disease [*I don't*], that diet is relevant in treating IBD.'

Startling, right? But a pretty common experience in the early noughties, and based on The National Institute for Health and Care Excellence (NICE) guidelines,[14] my doctor was right, and I would likely have the same conversation today.

Fortunately, I went ahead and ploughed my own furrow in the gluten-free wasteland – I was bucking a trend. It was hard going, but I persisted. Anytime I had a small amount of wheat, it reinforced my commitment to starting an elimination diet and following through.

*When we are unwell, we have the opportunity to get deeply interested in what makes us ill, even if those in authority don't necessarily support our instincts.*

Medical research is now starting to take the dietary elements of IBD seriously. There are leading teaching hospitals in the USA focusing on an anti-inflammatory diet for IBD.[15] We're going to explore some aspects of this later, but this isn't a diet book. No, it's a book about what healing your gut might look like for you.

Healing happens in many different ways, at many different levels in your body, mind and emotions. The information and practices you'll find here are designed to help you start your own unique exploration. To ask questions and compassionately support yourself, so you can examine what steps to take on your unique healing journey.

## Personalizing your gut knowledge

We are going to spend some time redefining your relationship with your gut. Yep, we will spend time getting more gut intelligent and way more gut compassionate than you could ever imagine possible. Right now, let's get back to irritation and inflammation, which is why you are here.

A key part of the jigsaw to managing your gut is creating a space to tune in mindfully to inflammation (*itis*) at its subtlest early stages. I've been fortunate to be well and generally symptom-free for 20 years (since my colon's near-miss with the scalpel), but what I have been doing pretty much consistently is showing up for my gut in the most loving, mindful and compassionate way I can. I've created a whole bunch of practices to help you lean into those early signs of *itis* and to start to recognize your body's triggers. These subtle, fluttering levels of discomfort are easy to ignore – and that's a problem.

For me, the *itis* scale starts with a subtle, unsettled feeling. You know when you can't quite put your finger on it? If I ignore those early *itis* fairies pulling at my gut, it moves towards a full, fizzing pain.

To capture those early signs, you need to slow down and show up for yourself using a few simple daily practices like the mindful base belly breathing practice, which I'll share in a moment. This is not airy-fairy stuff but deep biological processes that happen when you stop and breathe. In fact, this is all about your vagus nerve because what happens in vagus never just stays in vagus.

If I ignore the early signs and just rush on through, then sure as day follows night, the problem will grow: elevated C-reactive protein (CRP) levels, heat at the site of inflammation and a residue of low energy. Like a soluble aspirin in a glass of water, my blood vibrates. This *itis* builds up.

## Meet your gut with your breath

Begin by coming back to your breath. Not the usual city-shallow breathing but taking deep belly breaths to your base – your root and solar plexus chakras. These centres are particularly important for our gut health. The ancient Sanskrit word *chakra* means 'wheel' of energy originating from the Hindu/yoga tradition. You may already be familiar with the seven main energy centres that sit in a line at your core, from your root to the top of your head. They are interwoven with hundreds of subtler energy channels throughout the body.

Figure 4: Base belly breathing into the chakras

The breath can ground you deeply into your gut, right into the core of your being. Breathing with awareness reminds us we are embodied: body, heart and gut – all inextricably linked. There are many breathing

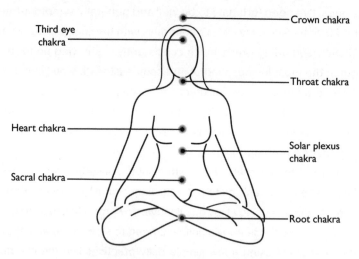

techniques you can explore that can help stimulate your vagus nerve and link you deeply into your parasympathetic nervous system. Below is a simple, portable little number, which I use daily.

## Base belly breathing

If you are going through an IBD flare right now, your breath can be a powerful healing agent to calm and support your gut. Spend three minutes doing this practice, then aim to take three breaths at least each hour – you can set a reminder on your phone. The aim is to slowly change the mindless habit of shallow breathing so that you are deeply in your body and belly. Once you've got this practice down pat, you can take it anywhere, anytime.

1. Find a quiet space and set a three-minute timer.
2. Sit upright comfortably with your back straight and your shoulders open. Place your non-dominant hand lightly on your belly, palm flat, and your dominant hand on your chest. Now take a deep breath into your lungs and imagine you are breathing deep into your root chakra (right into the base of your bum).
3. You will start to feel your non-dominant hand move outwards. As you naturally exhale your breath, imagine you are misting the glass of a mirror with your mouth slightly open. You can even make an 'ahh' sound.
4. Breathe in again and repeat. By focusing on drawing in your breath beyond your belly, down into your root chakra, you will naturally find you breathe more deeply. You will feel grounded and present.

*Note*: If this is the first time you've tried abdominal breathing, you may feel blocked. If this is the case, be gentle and take time to practise. If you continue to breathe deeply into your root chakra without forcing it, but calmly and with focus, you will find your energy shifts. This may be accompanied by an emotional shift. If you've received messages about it not being OK to cry or show emotion, you may notice a release in your diaphragm.

Many wisdom traditions recognize that the mind and body are connected through the breath. And you've just given your gut the simplest gift – a blessing of presence. The good news is you always have access to your breath. So, continue to notice your breath as you read on.

There is no traditional cure for IBD and IBS, but there is the ability to heal. You can take part in your unique dance with a compassionately empowered mindset. A mindset that transforms the way you relate to your gut. Deep at the core of your being, these secret organs sit in darkness, and the idea they are not working properly can feel overwhelming. You may feel that there is nothing that you can do about it. But you have already taken the first step and now know how the digestive tract works, so let's move on to the beautiful biology of your inner world.

## Gut Gaia

To make sense of how your body works, let's take a moment to scale this right up. In the 1970s, the philosopher James Lovelock envisioned the Gaia hypothesis.[16] In essence, he argued that planet Earth has its own internal system with delicate checks and balances to ensure its survival. Lovelock's work shifted old paradigms that conceived the planet as a vast land- and seascape, which could be plundered and exploited. This outdated world view is part of a destructive perspective contributing to extinction and damage to our planet Earth.

Over the last few decades, the Gaia concept has supported a shift in consciousness and greater global and environmental awareness. When Lovelock started to model the planet as inextricably impacted by humankind's actions, as vulnerable to damage, he created a model for us all. Something as simple as an idea can be powerful enough to shift our perspective.

Now let's take a step back to our human scale. Your body, like the planet, is always seeking homeostasis. For example, when we drink a glass of juice, the body produces insulin, stimulating the liver to store excess glucose in the form of glycogen.

*We, too, are like the planet Earth – carefully balanced, sensitive to a whole range of environmental factors that we place upon it.*

If we could shift our surface sense of ourselves, might this trigger a deeper personal revelation of our own internal workings? Are we each, in essence, our own Gaia? Before you complete the exercise below, take a look at this image of the small and large intestine.

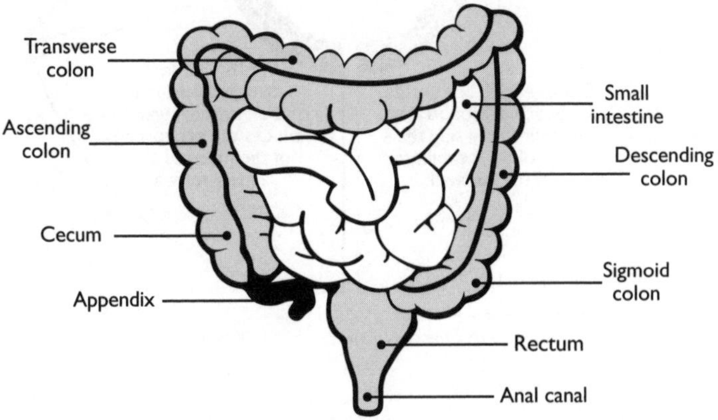


Figure 5: The small and large intestines

You know from Chapter 1 that your small intestine, with its three distinct sections (the duodenum, jejunum and ileum), is a long sausage-like tube, while your large intestine is shorter and fatter with kinks and consists of the cecum and rectum. All too often, our gut is an underpaid sweatshop worker, enduring pretty impossible working conditions. These sensitive organs toil in darkness whilst we, the careless boss, add extra pressure by mindlessly consuming the wrong stuff. If you have damaged villi due to chronic inflammation, this can lead to a vicious cycle, which increases inflammation.

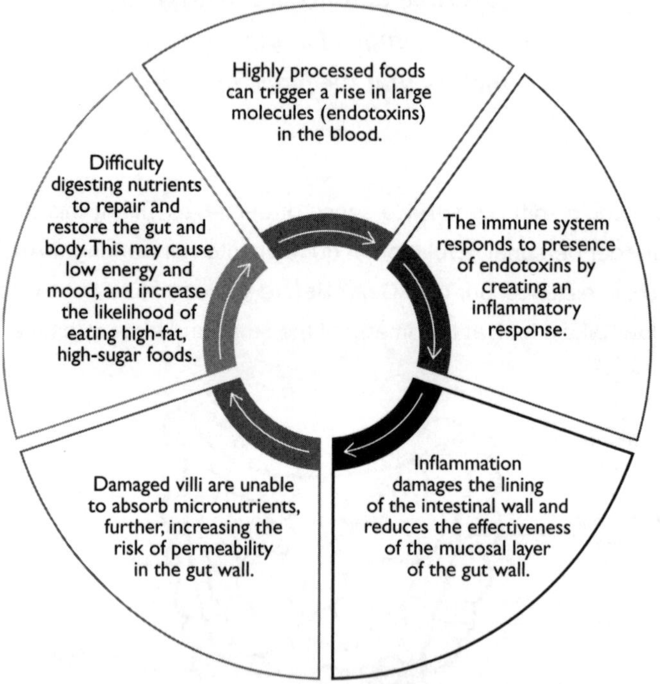


Figure 6: The cycle of chronic inflammation

The fact that most of us have a pretty thoughtless relationship with our inner digestive world is understandable – it's hidden away out of sight and out of mind. But deep in the dark recesses of our guts, we pay the price with our wellbeing.

## *Liberate your gut with kindness.*

Once you've started to cultivate compassion for your colon, you'll find you're more motivated to do right by each of the microscopic pink fingers of your villi. How do we keep them well and healthy?

Pause for a moment, take a breath and consider your dear gut. I encourage you to breathe deeply into your belly as you learned in the base belly breathing exercise (*see page 31*). This time, however, I'd like you to go a little deeper with the following exercise. This practice will be especially helpful if you have a flare right now and it's important that you approach your inner environment with tenderness and compassion. These inner organs work tirelessly for you, even when you are unwell.

## Gut Gaia visualization

You can get a friend or partner to read this to you or even record it and follow the visualization at your own pace and have your Gut-loving Journal to hand.

1. Find a comfortable place to sit or preferably lie down and spend a few minutes taking seven deep base belly breaths (*see page 31*).

2. Start by imagining you are shrinking until you are so tiny you can climb into your mouth. In *Inner Space*, one of my favourite films from the 80s, Dennis Quaid did just that.

3. Go past your teeth, slip between the salivary glands – the first part of your digestive system. If you gulp down your food and barely chew it properly, you'll cause more pressure later in the digestive system.

4. Now move down the oesophagus, the first part of your digestive tract.

5. Your stomach is churning and processing your last meal – that slice of rye and the coffee you gulped back earlier. It's pretty acidic here, with a pH of 1.5–3.5, and mucus protects the stomach walls.

6. Rest here for a moment, look around at the colours, shapes. What can you hear? You'll notice little waves releasing fluid into your duodenum. You might see poorly chewed, oversized food particles.

7. Take a close look at the wall of your ileum. You'll notice the lining is covered in tiny finger-like villi. These fingers increase the surface area, supporting your ileum to extract nutrients from your food. They feed a rich tapestry of interwoven capillaries, which enter your bloodstream. Can you see darker patterns of dark, red, inflamed ileum, little scars of old battles? If you have Crohn's disease, you may want to spend a little longer here.

8. Trust your gut to guide you. Examine the thin single-layer cells of the plicae circulares (tiny crypts in the folds of your gut wall) – are they looking pink and healthy? Or does your duodenum despair as yet more sugar and gluten swim out of your stomach? Can you see you see your immune cells getting stuck in, trying to mop up the mess?

9. You are travelling to the centre of your gut. Let's keep going further. The end of the ileum leads to your large intestine – the colon.

10. How are the walls of your colon looking? Smooth, pink and happy, or darkened and swollen? Take a closer look. Can you see deforested patches of villi, sites of damage? You may even find places where the passageway is narrowed and thickened by scars from past 'flare-ups'.

11. Stay in the colon for few moments, especially if you have ulcerative colitis, and send healing love and light. The tender single-layer lining of the gut is more delicate than the eye's cornea, and a healthy gut replaces this single layer every three days.

12. When you feel you have completed your journey, say thank you to your guts and tell them you'll see them again soon. Come back to your full-size body and exhale deeply. Spend a little time writing your reflections in your Gut-loving Journal.

*Your body is always ready to heal and recover if you give it the right conditions. Gut knowledge to gut healing is a process.*

## Your gut story

Let's admit it, most of us like quick fixes and simple solutions. In fact, I bet right now, you would be happy to pop a pill and continue right on with your life, just the way you are. Right?

Unfortunately, most meds for gut health (not all) work by suppressing symptoms. Stop the meds, and the symptoms return. So whilst taking medication may be an essential part of your treatment plan (and I would never advocate stopping prescribed meds), they don't get to the root cause of the inflammation and irritability at the heart of your gut health problems.

The big picture is complex. In medical terminology, it's 'multifactorial'. Doctors don't yet fully understand all the different factors that contribute to gut health problems. Still, the picture *is* getting pretty interesting, primarily because of the exciting research on the microbiome.

In our modern hand-sanitizing obsessed world, we generally look down on bugs as things to purge and purify. Meaning it's all too easy to discount the 100 trillion bugs in your gut. Of course, they are tiny, invisible and many don't even have a name. They have survived because they play a crucial role in humankind's survival. Our story is intimately interwoven with these bugs; they shape many aspects of our physical health, and the evidence is increasingly pointing to their role in our mental health.[17] In fact, the picture starting to emerge is:

> *[The] microbes in our gut may even influence our behaviour and the way we think. Studies in animals show that the range of microbes in their gut can influence their resilience to anxiety and stress.*[18]

The factors that shape the health and balance of our microbiome are wide-ranging. Some of them start before we are born; exposure to antibiotics during pregnancy and whether we were born via a natural or caesarean delivery can impact the diversity of our microbiome as a baby.[19] Breastfeeding also gives our microbiome a head start by training our immune system and pre-populating our good gut bugs.[20] Antibiotics in the first years of life, exposure to environmental pollutants and where you grew up all shape the range and diversity of your gut fauna, so let's take a closer look at your gut story.

This is all about looking back, so you can see forwards. The exercise below may take a little time and detective work. So, let's deepen the gut narrative:

- to understand how you and your gut got to where you are right now: flare, remission, bloat or pain
- to bear witness to your personal gut journey

This is your chance to gather up your own gut tale thread by thread.

## Get to know your gut story

Choose a quiet space. Block out a morning or afternoon in your diary and commit. You'll need some paper, if possible, at least 10 large pieces and different-colour pens. Spread out the paper across the floor of your room. Each sheet of paper represents a step in your gut story. Start with your pre-birth if you can access this. If not, start from as early as you can, and work right up to today and include gut health facts, general wellbeing, family and home life, study, work.

**Pre-birth gut story:** Pregnancy complications, food cravings (you may need to interview your mum or dad here if that's possible). Did your mum have any antibiotic treatment during pregnancy?

**Birth:** C-section or vaginal delivery, complications, induced, early, late, antibiotics or drugs during the process.

**Age 0–12 months:** Your first year, medical interventions, home-life events, illnesses or infections, colic or distress with food, breastfeeding, etc.

**Age 1–5 years:** Preschool nursery, illnesses, diet, food allergies, courses of antibiotics, etc.

**Age 5–11 years:** Oral health. What did you eat for breakfast? What were your favourite foods? What was your school canteen like?

**Age 12–16 years:** This is when you may have become body-conscious and dieting and food fads can be most evident. What were yours? How did this impact your gut and your microbiome? What bacteria were you cooking up in your biome?

**Age 17–21 years:** Alcohol is inflammatory, so if there was a certain point where you started drinking heavily in your teens, put that down. Or if there were a few incidences of binge drinking, get that down. You may start to track changes. If you moved away from home, how was your diet? What did you eat?

**First symptoms:** In the 12 months before symptoms, note your stress levels, environmental changes, family, home and work life, studies, a holiday to a foreign climate.

**Diagnosis:** It's pretty normal to have several trips to your GP with different symptoms before you get an accurate diagnosis. In fact, it can take some time for the right diagnosis.

**Response to medication:** What worked? Any relapses?

**Anything else:** You can add steps depending on the story of your symptoms.

Now review your sheets of paper in turn by walking your line. As you walk, enter into the time that you and your gut were experiencing. To help you, ask the following questions:

- How do I feel now?
- How's my gut feeling right now?

You can travel up and down your gut story timeline. If you need to go back and revisit anything, add in detail. But I suggest starting at your birth and work to the present day. Write down your feelings and thoughts at each stage on the paper.

It's important to have thinking time. This is a space for you to commune with your gut. Try and speak in the present tense, journeying along the tract of your gut. What sights, sounds, smells and, above all, feelings did you experience? Once you have the full picture of your gut story, or as full as you can make it, you can take stock and zone in on the specifics.

- Has your gut had some specific shocks? Repeated courses of antibiotics in childhood can wreak havoc on the delicate balance of a toddler's microbiome.
- Have you experienced a bout of food poisoning at a critical time in your gut story? How does that link to your symptoms?

Gather up your pieces of paper and place them inside your Gut-loving Journal. Keep adding to any part of your story as you learn more and start joining up your gut story's dots.

Using this exercise, you'll start to build the unique foundation of your gut knowledge and be able to rewrite it into a more gut-loving story. In terms of the causes of gut health issues, there are elements you can't control: your genes, your parents' (yep, your mum *and* dad) pre-pregnancy diet and your exposure to childhood pollutants, which may predispose you to gut health problems. But you do have some influence on your epigenetics. Epigenetics explores how your inherited genes get switched on or off by your environment and behaviour. Imagine your inherited DNA is a bit like a family cookbook packed full of recipes. Your personal epigenetics are like the notes in the margins. You get to decide on how to tweak the flavours, swap out ingredients and change the meal. What notes do you have in the margins of your unique recipe book? Geneticist Dr Adam Rutherford says, 'Our microbial makeup depends on our medical history, our location and our diet. It's a signature that can be very different to even our closest relatives.'[21]

Environmental factors are always shaping and interacting with our genes – stress, diet, smoking, alcohol, lifestyle all shape our health. What we do know is there's *something* about Western city living that's pretty bad for our guts.

OK, so you've started to explore your micro-environment and your beautiful microbiome. Let's go a little deeper still and rewrite our gut story.

CHAPTER 3

# REWRITING YOUR GUT STORY

*'Your story is what you have, what you will always have. It is something to own.'*

MICHELLE OBAMA, AUTHOR AND FORMER FIRST LADY OF THE USA

Using the Gut Gaia visualization (*see page 35*) and gut story exercise (*see page 38*) will help you get to the root of any disconnect between your knowledge and actions. To join the dots and help you make sense of where you are. When you don't really see what's going on, you may be causing your already troubled guts more problems. In this chapter, we're going to explore what keeps us stuck in unhealthy gut habits and the often-unconscious gut stories we tell ourselves. We'll also explore our wider family food values and how they show up in how we choose to eat. I think you know what I mean, but let me tell you a story.

In my twenties, I backpacked across the east coast of the USA with my best friend, Helen. I loved it, and one of my fondest memories is sitting in the big train stations of New York and Boston, where I'd grab a coffee and a pretzel. The Auntie Anne's pretzel stand with its blue gingham awning was distinctive and wholesome. Whenever we passed through, I'd smell those sweet carbs and go get one – my favourite was cinnamon and sugar. I would eat that pretzel, and hey presto, an hour later I would have pretzel-bloat. The next day, I'd promise myself *no more pretzel eating*, and then before the end of the day, I'd have a big, pretzel-bloated belly and beat myself up.

Sound familiar?

Well, I was astonished to learn that some of this is because I was an addict. The bad bacteria in my gut were calling out for the highly processed, sugar-filled fat molecules. We now know that if you have sensitivity to gluten and dairy, your body will create morphine-like chemicals gluteomorphin and casomorphin. In a bizarre twist, these chemicals give you a natural high. You may even feel a pleasurable dulling dopamine effect after your favourite food.

My husband, David, is a true cheese lover – cheddar, blue, brie, you name it he loves it, and over time (and, well, maybe because he is married to a crazy gut-loving lady), he's noticed a pattern of brain fog and tiredness after a cheese plate. Maybe you've found foods that trigger a similar response in you? And, if you've noticed that reaction, do you still eat your favourite food? Well, I'm guessing, yes, sometimes you do. Why?

## Trigger foods and gut dysbiosis

The answer to that is a little complex, and you need to explore your personal gut psychology and biology to get to the root. In *10% Human*, Alanna Collen[22] explains how we have co-evolved with the 2kg (4lb 7oz) of bacteria in our gut, our microbiome. When we regularly eat highly processed, refined high-sugar foods, we feed the gut's unhelpful microbes. Ironically it's the foods we are intolerant to that we often feel most addicted to. So, on top of the morphine-like chemicals our inflamed gut is producing, we also have our microbes to consider.

Eating your trigger foods repeatedly may provide an important part of the jigsaw for your gut trouble. When you feed the unfriendly gut bacteria, you can also create an imbalance in your gut microbiome known as dysbiosis.

Dysbiosis can be triggered by a range of things. As adults, some of the common triggers are excessive alcohol, extended periods of poor sleep (disruption in the circadian rhythm, our inner body clock, that supports our waking and sleep cycle) or frequent antibiotics courses. We and our inner bugs are co-living and co-evolving. Our inner microbiome is a finely tuned environment, and when we regularly eat junk food, we are in effect growing our own inner addicts.

*The more highly processed foods you eat, the more you – and the more destructive army of inner hitchhikers in your gut – crave those high-sugar, refined foods.*

So yes, your microbes are shaped by what you eat. Your food can feed the good bugs or the less helpful ones. But there's another level to this. Right now, for most of us, our gorgeous inner workers, our microscopic villi, our ileum, the beautifully balanced world of our microbes, are not real. They're hidden away behind skin and fat – out of sight and out of mind. Even our best intentions get forgotten if we can't see the consequences. I know that disconnect because I've been there – so many times.

## Why do we hurt ourselves with food?

Sometimes in those moments, it's easier, maybe, to eat what the kids are eating, not to be a fussy house guest – or you've had a tough day and that extra level of 'self-discipline' makes you feel like you're missing out. Why shouldn't you just have a little slice of that birthday cake? Sometimes that fluffy, light, wheaty food is going to call you.

I'm a sucker for the little free biscotti on my coffee saucer and the smell of freshly toasted bread. Forbidden pastries have got my number – a crisp, buttery croissant or pain au chocolat. They shout out to you across the bakery counter, blast into your unsuspecting nostrils as you pop to check out the small section of the 'free from' aisle at your local supermarket. Starting a gluten-free or dairy-free journey can be tough, but let's just get this whole thing into perspective. You have a choice, and that choice is made up of a thousand smaller daily choices.

## *Food values*

So loud and proud – food is a factor in your gut health. Food shapes your life; it's a key driver. For most of us, our relationship with food is a little complicated. Food is family, food is comfort, leisure and pleasure all rolled into one. Food reveals so much about our fundamental identity values (plant-based, pescatarian, meat and two veg); our aspirations (paleo or low FODMAP); and, of course, our heritage (Italian, Irish, Indian).

If you're sitting on the cusp of making conscious changes to how you eat, you have to acknowledge the sheer complexity of these often-unconscious drivers – all of them shape your relationship to food. The way you relate to your plate is built on habit. Deep, often unconscious, patterns. Gut health problems can be a wake-up call, a time to unravel your behaviours and reframe your automatic approach to food. This is your chance to start to reframe your personal food story.

## *Family food stories*

Your personal story is inevitably tied up in a larger context; family, culture and human. For the first time in history, more people are dying from overeating than undereating. Let's just take a minute to digest that. It turns out that some of the worst bits of the standard Western diet are wreaking havoc on our gut. Now, like everything, it's complicated. But whatever your situation, the food you put in your body contributes to your gut health.

In this next exercise, you're going to explore family food heritage. Your family food culture becomes your 'norm'. It's a kind of baseline that you operate from. So, getting familiar with that baseline and how it has shaped your family and your personal gut health is a key part of understanding and rewriting your own gut story.

You might just be surprised where this conversation takes you. Go there.

## Family foods

Have a 'food conversation' with your oldest living relative first and then other members of your family. Approach this task with curiosity. And hey, who doesn't like to talk about food. Here are a few starting questions:

- What did you eat for breakfast/lunch/dinner? Where did you eat? What time?
- What did you eat on special occasions/birthdays/religious festivals/weekends?
- How about favourite/hated/forbidden foods?

Listen to the emotion behind the words, the images, tastes and smells. The conversation will likely take an unexpected turn to two – go with it. Take your phone and record if you can; this is the oral history of your family. You're creating a kind of living food jigsaw as each conversation fills in a different part.

Now that you have more context, go a little deeper into your personal relationship with food. It's the very predictability of childhood foods that can make them feel like a 'safe haven', particularly at times of uncertainty.

When our brains are wired up and overstimulated, familiar foods are quite literally a no-brainer. So many familiar neural pathways lead us right back to where we started. As a child of the 80s, I had a fair few sugary sweets and salty, skinny fries feeding my particular gut bugs – and I've spent the last decade trying to starve them out. The more gut-loving information I learn, the easier it gets. Leading plant-based advocate Dr Michael Gregor suggests, 'The primary reason diseases tend to run in families may be that diets tend to run in families.'[23] That's certainly food for thought. Time to direct your gaze within and look at what you've been feeding your microbes.

## Food iceberg

Approach this exercise with gentle gut care because this is how you can start to lovingly unstick yourself and your gut. So, how do you show up to your plate?

Think about food as your personal food iceberg. The bit above the water is your conscious choices around food, but there's usually a whole lot happening below the waterline. You're going to gently bring awareness to those bits by noting down your answers to the following questions:

- What are your strongest food memories?
- What foods do you feel you cannot live without? (It's amazing how often I hear cheese in this category. Thank you, casomorphins. These little darlings can attach to dopamine receptors in the brain when you eat dairy.)[24]
- What are your comfort foods? What are your taboo foods? What foods do you want to squirrel away when times are scarce?

Once you see your belief that you, for example, 'simply can't live without pasta' and it is all about your Italian grandmother's homemade lasagne – a dish you associate with being nurtured as a child – you understand it for what it is. A lovely memory that may or may not serve your gut health today.

From this exercise, take a bit of time to journal your own food memories and associations – a space to start to make sense of your food phobias and addictions and the rest in between.

What you might start to notice are those 'screw it' moments. When you just want to eat, it often focuses on your trigger foods. In Part II, I'll share some strategies for dealing with these triggers.

OK, now you have a gutful of self-awareness, you'll notice your triggers and those habits towards comfort foods that don't serve you or your gut. So, time to set some goals.

# Chapter 4

# Setting Healthy Gut Goals

*'Between stimulus and response, there is a space. In that space is our power to choose our response. In our response lies our growth and our freedom.'*

Victor Frankl, *Man's Search for Meaning*

Even small changes have the potential to take us to a remarkably different place. We tend to shuttle along the same tracks of habit and familiarity. But we always have the option to pivot – even a little – in a healing direction, and that can lead to remarkable results. I know. I'm living that change.

## Changing up your habits

How long it takes you to replace an old habit and create a new one depends on your motivation and consistency. The key to sustaining transformation is to focus on accumulating small changes over time. And each moment, you get to choose your journey.

*'People who want to kick their habit for reasons that are aligned with their personal values will change their behaviour faster than people who are doing it for external reasons...'*

ELLIOT BERKMAN PHD[25]

This is about waking up to every moment of your life and getting familiar with the building blocks of habits: why you choose the foods you buy, what you cook and how you eat. That's a pretty fundamental root-and-branch change right there. Having a goal – a really clear goal – is the keystone to success, so it's time to think about yours.

## Gut health vision

Whatever the state of your gut health right at this moment, I encourage you to get sensory. There's a certain magic in visualizing, hearing, feeling, smelling, even tasting your goal. To move forwards, you need to get compassionately clear, so take out your Gut-loving Journal and think about the following questions:

- What aspiration do you have for your gut health?
- In a gut-healthy life, how would your day start?
- What food would you choose for breakfast?
- How far are you away from that right now?
- What is your motivation for change?

OK, there's power in that vision. Jot it down. We're going to come back to it later. My personal wake-up call (and I've had a few) was my growing understanding of what chronic background inflammation does to the body. Inflammation is bad for your WHOLE system – heart, brain and gut.

As I already mentioned, I was told by a well-qualified, well-intentioned doctor that wheat wasn't a factor for me as inflammation was busily ravaging my colon. The simple truth was my whole body told me it was, so I listened to my gut wisdom. And, just for the record, I don't think I would be sitting here today with my colon if I hadn't listened.

Just as we are each unique, so too is our microbiome. Therefore, the ulcerative colitis I experience isn't your ulcerative colitis. Our bodies get ill for different reasons, and we often heal in different ways. I found a part of my healing journey in my food choices, but it's more than what we eat. Food matters, but it's also how we live our lives. The body keeps count. So how do you tune in to your own innate wisdom?

## Using your growing gut knowledge for change

Using your gut knowledge is a process of moving against a tide of easy-access foods. I'm not going to lie to you; it isn't always easy. There are two aspects to changing your diet. The obvious one is the **cost**. Sometimes healthy foods cost more. Processed, high-sugar, high-fat foods are cheap, easy fuel. The second is **time**. If you are time-poor – and let's face it, most of us are – eating healthily can feel difficult. I want to be honest and upfront about that. It's the simple truth that healthy food usually takes more planning and preparation than less healthy convenience foods.

I share some of my simple go-to recipes in Part V, but as quick and easy as they are, they are not microwave meals. They are gut-loving, mindful foods. Food is all about the inner and outer Gaia. The meals I make are mindful, gut-fully prepared to love your belly, and love the belly of the world. It's the kind of food where we ask:

- What am I feeding my gut bugs today?
- How will this food make me feel?

I love these questions. They can tune us right back in to our inner ecosystem because...

*Feeding our dear gut bugs with diverse goodness matters.*

## Magical microbiome

So, let's get a bit technical again, as we're all about **gut-loving knowledge**. What's really fascinating about our microbiome's beautiful world is that we don't fully understand it yet. Like a new galaxy, we are just starting to map out the pattern of stars and, remember, we haven't even named them all.

The extent of the microbiome's involvement in our health is staggering. So far, 29 different health conditions have been linked to a lack of diversity or an imbalance in the microbiome. Here's betting this list is going to get longer. It includes type 2 diabetes, high cholesterol, heart failure, renal failure and osteoarthritis, according to genome analysis of more than 400,000 individuals presented at the European Society of Cardiology:

> *It is becoming increasingly clear that an individual's gut microbiome composition, which is defined by both genetic and environmental factors such as diet, may affect his/her susceptibility to certain diseases....*[26]

There is a world within you just as exciting as any Netflix miniseries. Imagine all those battles for dominion, struggles to find food, tales of reproduction amongst thousands of different bacteria species. Some bacteria are great in moderation. Others, like salmonella and E.coli, are out-and-out dangerous to human health.

We know that an imbalance in our microbiome may well impact the integrity of our single-celled gut wall,[27] and some of the most common triggers for dysbiosis are worth reminding ourselves about: antibiotics, stress, poor diet, exposure to chemical pollutants, excess alcohol. Twin those with genetic predisposition, and we have compromised gut health.[28]

As scientists map the human microbiome, we learn more about the weird and wonderful world hidden in the gut, and research is alive and kicking around the biome and IBD. In the UK and USA, there are now a few ways you get your biome mapped.

### ♥ Gut Love ♥

The more we engage in gut research, the more we can map the human gut biome, and see how tending to our gut bugs contributes to a wider *stewardship* of the global human microbiome[29]. I have mapped my microbiome; it's a great way to get a good snapshot of our internal ecosystem and to become custodian of our gut bugs.

Let's take a closer look at a few of the key players in the microbiome. What's emerging is that those of us with IBD tend to have an overpopulation of less friendly gut bugs while having a shortage of good gut bugs.[30] In fact, there are particular patterns of over- and underpopulation of different bacteria in Crohn's disease and ulcerative colitis, depending on the site of inflammation. The key messages are diversity, and also about the 3Ps: probiotics, prebiotics and polyphenols. We'll have a more detailed look at the 3Ps in Part III, and you'll find some recipes in Part V.

For IBS symptoms, where bloating and discomfort predominate, there is evidence that eating foods like live-cultured yoghurt, kefir and miso can increase our lovely **lactobacillus gut bugs**. You've probably heard of them – one of the best known of the friendly bacteria found in many probiotic drinks and supplements. Bonus – there's also evidence lactobacillus helps support our mental health. So it's certainly a gut bug to nurture if, like me, you have IBS or IBD with IBS overlay.

*Take supplements but remember they won't counteract a poor diet. Remember your food choices; feed your microbes.*

Our aim in gut health is always to create an anti-inflammatory environment. So you want to increase the super friendly bifidobacteria – these little bugs help break down complex carbohydrates in your gut. If you are a cheese eater, you may have plenty of this. For plant-based diets, try out fermented goodies and inulin-rich chicory and artichoke. Bacteroidetes[31] also help reduce inflammation. These lovely gut bugs will help you to maintain a healthy weight. They are great at breaking down the undigested fibre in vegetables and supporting your immune system.

## It's all about the butyrate

While the scientists are still unravelling the actual bacteria patterns in different forms of Crohn's disease and ulcerative colitis, what's clear is we want to help the bugs that counteract gut inflammation. Butyrate feeds the cells that line the gut wall. It's not quite as simple as eating butyrate (although there are high levels of it in high-fat foods like butter and olive oil). You can support your gut bugs to create butyrate by increasing the foods they like to eat: apples, garlic, chickpeas, kiwi and almonds.

And there's a little aside here. Be careful about restricted diets low in carbs and fibre as they can actually impair your body's butyrate production. Hence why long periods on the low FODMAP diet (one of the central treatment protocols for IBS) are not recommended, as this diet excludes some important gut-healing foods.

When you rest and reset your digestive system by an occasional seasonal fast or a later breakfast, we help our amazing **Akkermansia** flourish. This little bug lives on the mucus lining of the bowel and acts to strengthen the gut wall and reduce inflammation (potentially reducing the risk of diabetes and obesity).[32] Simply aiming to give your guts a little restorative rest for 14 hours, or even 15–16 hours, allows it to flourish. For me, this is seasonal; I tend to eat a warming earlier breakfast in the colder months. So go with your gut on this. If fasting isn't your thing, try adding a handful of organic cranberries to your morning porridge.

The beautiful **Roseburia** bacteria is another one of the good girls in the gut. I have high levels, which may in part explain my long period of remission from ulcerative colitis symptoms. Roseburia bacteria thrive when fed with the 3Ps – a probiotic-, prebiotic- and polyphenol-rich diet.

**Barnesiella** is definitely a gut bug you want to cultivate if you have IBD or IBS, and it has been shown to have anti-inflammatory effects in mice. It has some amazing properties in humans, including reducing the risk of antibiotic-resistant bugs in the gut.[33]

OK, that's just a little snapshot. More and more information is being published around our biome each week. So, tune in and grow that gut-loving knowledge. I've included some Resources for those gut geeks that want to get deeper into this.

If you want to protect your gut health, then avoid emulsifiers like mono- and diglycerides. These are commonly used as food additives and small quantities are often added to packaged foods to extend shelf life. But remember, what's good for food manufacturers' profit margins is rarely good for our waistlines or our guts. We'll take a closer look at this in Parts II and III.

OK, what a journey that's been. Let's take stock and reflect, so get out your Gut-loving Journal for the final exercise in this chapter.

## Gut life letter

Now you've comprehensively watered the seeds of your new gut knowledge, take a moment to tune in to your gut wisdom.

1. Start with a clear intention and be open to hearing what your gut needs to tell you.
2. Breathe in and hold your belly, say in a loving voice, 'Precious Gut, how you are? I'm listening.'
3. Then, taking up your pen, write and let it flow naturally, unedited, to capture that inner gut voice.

---

As we end Part I, continue to read widely, commit wholeheartedly to building your gut knowledge and follow your gut instinct. This is your body, your life and your gut.

*Remember: You are wise – you contain multitudes.*

## GUT KNOWLEDGE

- Keep reflecting on your personal gut story and how you can change your gut narrative (*see page 37*).
- Practice tuning in to your personal gut knowledge through journalling and visualization (*see pages 19 and 35*).
- Discover more about your personal gut microbiome (*see page 54*).
- Start nourishing your gut bugs (*see pages 55–57*).

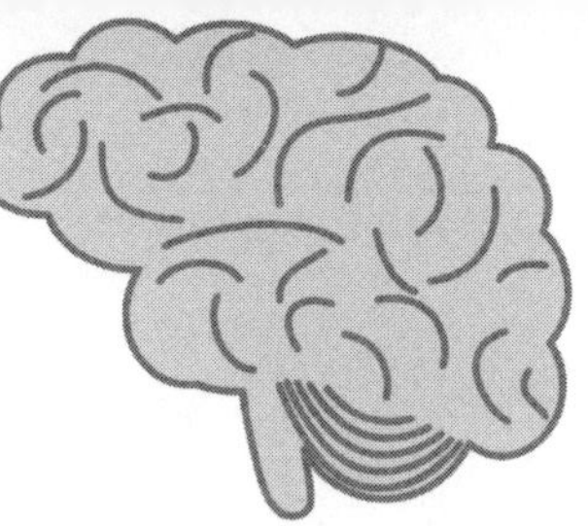

# Part II

# GUT COMPASSION

***'With self-compassion, we give ourselves the same kindness and care we'd give to a good friend.'***

Dr Kristin Neff, expert and author on self-compassion

Self-compassion is the bridge between what we know and what we do, and in Part II, we're getting gut compassionate. We'll look at the impact of the standard Western diet and lifestyle on anxiety and mental health. We'll shine a light onto the gut-wrenching emotions we so unconsciously hold in our bloated, unhappy bellies. And we'll delve deeper into journalling and strategies that can release old emotional habits.

You'll discover how your gut-fierce compassion can deepen your own gut instinct and lead to a more mindful approach to shopping and eating. Finally, I'll share a few practical ways to better care for your gut, with gut-loving massage and yoga for sleep.

What you'll discover over and over is that compassion is the bridge between your new gut knowledge and more healthy gut-led life choices.

## CHAPTER 5

# THE ANXIOUS GUT

*'Untangle the knot, Soften the glare.*
*Settle your dust.'*

LAO TZU, SIXTH-CENTURY CHINESE PHILOSOPHER

I'm guessing you know all about the anxious gut, right? The anxious gut is fed by cortisol straight from the adrenal glands. That familiar soundtrack of fight or flight triggers the amygdala – part of the ancient brain. This response happens in microseconds before we are consciously aware of potential danger.[1] It's when the amygdala hijacks your brain that you are triggered into strong reactive emotions like anxiety, fear and anger. The anxious gut is the place of overwhelm.

You know how it goes: the cycle of anxiety is on repeat: long commutes, work presentations, buzzing phones – they all play havoc with our ancient brain. Our hyperstimulated stress system loads our anxious, bloated bellies. The gut is where emotions can get stuck, and there's an increasingly strong link between gut health and mental health. So the foods we'll explore in Parts II and III are not only gut-healing but reduce anxiety.

## Healing self-compassion

I'm so excited to see recent studies showing what, at some level, my gut instinct always told me. Self-compassion reduces inflammation in the body.[2] This hasn't been looked at specifically in IBD, but scientists have studied inflammatory markers in the body.

One recent study found that higher levels of compassion, wisdom and social support are linked to a richer, more diverse gut microbiome. The opposite is also true, folks – lower levels of compassion and social connectedness are linked to reduced microbial diversity.

Tanya T. Nguyen PhD, assistant professor of psychiatry at UC San Diego School of Medicine, said that 'the mechanisms that may link loneliness, compassion and wisdom with gut microbial diversity are not known, but observed reduced microbial diversity typically represents worse physical and mental health.'[3]

Fascinating stuff, right?

And when we talk about stress, we think it is 'all in our head', and the problem with that way of thinking is we forget that stress is real. It has its own chemistry. Stress has specific, measurable biological impacts on the body and what's significant is that it appears to work both ways. Stress increases the likelihood of inflammation and vice versa.[4]

The next time you're exasperated or tough on yourself for feeling stressed, remember it's not just in your head. Do you want lower blood pressure, improved digestion, less anxiety and greater resilience? Well, think back to what you learned about the vagus nerve in Part I because you may need to aim to increase your vagal tone. Low vagal tone is associated with a range of health problems: stress and anxiety, poor gut health and lack of gut bug diversity. Too much sitting, poor sleep and an out of sync circadian rhythm, even smoking or excessive alcohol all appear to be implicated in reduced vagal tone. So how can you get that vagus toned right up?

## ♥ Gut Love ♥

Higher vagal tone increases mental resilience, meaning the body can relax faster after high-stress situations. Some simple ways to get toned include:

- Breathwork – a few deep base belly breaths (*see page 31*) will tone your vagus nerve and shift you into your parasympathetic nervous system (rest and repair setting).
- Practise intermittent fasting by having a later breakfast and early dinner so that you give your digestive system a little R&R. (*see page 132*).
- Take probiotics (*see pages 137–138*).
- Do mindfulness and loving-kindness practices, like the ones I share in this chapter, including visualization exercises.[5]
- Splash your face with cold water. If you are brave, go for a full-blast cold shower. Breathe deeply and relax as you do this.
- Have a hug for at least 30 seconds and combine with a few deep breaths. If there's no one to hug, then try self-soothing by using the havening technique, a simple exercise to put you into a 'safe space' and reduce stress (*see Resources, page 263*).
- Do a yoga stretch. Cobra is a wonderful way to stimulate the vagus nerve in the neck and deepen vagal stimulation combined with base belly breathing (*see Resources, page 263*).
- Sing, hum or chant out some gut-loving affirmations (*see page 151*).
- Massage, self-massage or a foot rub from a loved one (*see page 103*).

- Exercise in all its shapes and forms.
- Laughing and socializing (but go easy on the alcohol).
- Practise Gut Love Dance – a fun, soulful way of connecting to your gut through mindful movement. We'll take a look at how to create your very own dance in Part III.

Still feeling stressed or anxious? Well, new models are emerging, which can help us reframe our response to heightened feelings. In the book *How Emotions are Made*,[6] Dr Lisa Feldman Barrett explores how to reframe your stress response by being aware and simply renaming it. This approach can be particularly helpful for short-term triggers. Rather than name the flood of cortisol as 'terror' at a big presentation, you recognize you have a choice to reframe the 'stress trigger' as 'excitement' and the motivation to do well. I like this positive take on stress. However, if you're stuck in repeated patterns of fear or stress response, you'll need to be skilful in finding new ways to reframe new mindful habits. At these times of feeling most stuck in a repeated pattern, you may need to take yourself and your gut by the hand. Get into your body, breathe and ask:

- What are my choices right now?
- What am I assuming?
- How does this habit serve me, and what does it cost?
- What can this situation teach me?

As you ask these questions, you may start to feel a subtle shift in your ways of being. All these techniques can help to shift your automatic ways of operating in the world.

## How's my anxious gut doing today?

The habit of anxiety can feel hard-wired, an old pattern that seems stuck on rinse and repeat. And if that's the case, try to place your personal anxiety in context because the real story is that anxiety levels are high. And, well, I don't know about you, but in an increasingly fluid and complex world, anxiety makes a kind of sense. Much of the research to understand the growth of anxiety and depression disorders focuses on social expectations and social media. But we can also look closer to home. At what we are eating.

Professor Felice Jacka has analysed wide-ranging data showing high levels of junk food are linked with an increased risk of depression and anxiety.[7] Leading scientists Professors Bonnie Kaplan and Julia Rucklidge's longitudinal studies demonstrate that plant-based diets higher in whole foods, nuts, good oils and fish are consistently associated with a lower risk of these mental health challenges.[8] The evidence is clear: your dietary intake today is a major determinant of your mental health in the future. To understand how diet can impact brain health and practical steps you can take to improve your diet, I recommend reading Rucklidge and Kaplan's book *The Better Brain* .

## The gut–mind relationship

We are still understanding all the complex ways our inner gut bugs shape our behaviour and mood. But what is clear is that the bugs in our gut contribute to our mood and mental state. Take, for example, the studies that demonstrate transplanting poop from depressed humans can cause animals to become depressed.[9] OK, this may sound a little yucky! But the transplantation of poop is the easiest way to package our unique set of individual gut bugs. Human studies have shown some exciting outcomes in managing Clostridium difficile infection[10] and are currently being rolled out for large-scale randomized trials to treat IBD.

So our gut bugs shape how we feel. And whilst we are still getting a clearer picture of exactly how this mechanism works and the specific bacteria involved, we know that it's the diversity and range of bacteria that are key to a balanced biome. We know that our gut produces around 90 per cent of our feel-good, anti-anxiety hormone serotonin. Serotonin not only improves mood but also supports gastrointestinal motility.

Our gut bugs also produce around 50 per cent of our dopamine levels.[11] Now dopamine is a big deal for our mood regulation, and it appears keeping our gut bugs healthy and diverse can support our production of a wide range of key neurotransmitters, which impact behaviour and mood.

What's beginning to emerge is the cycle of health issues caused by an inflamed and imbalanced gut. Those of us with a predisposition to gut health problems and who consume a high proportion of processed food may inadvertently reprogramme our gut for trouble. And once the balance of bacteria has been tipped into an unhealthy one, we get stuck in a kind of inflammatory cycle.

This cycle develops into low energy and low mood, then we crave the sweet stuff, alcohol and foods which give us a superficial boost, and of course, our very cravings are egged on by our inner gut bugs quite literally wanting to consume the high fat and sugar content of so many processed foods.

Once begun, this cycle can be hard to escape. But the key is, when you start to really understand what's occurring, you can halt the cycle and reclaim your gorgeous gut and re-establish a healthier, more balanced inner ecosystem.

Studies in mice found that eating a junk-food diet can act to reprogramme their immune system, in effect making it trigger-happy and more likely to produce inflammation and overreact to even minor stimuli with an overactive inflammatory response.[12]

Sound familiar? Well, as someone who has lived for 20 years with IBD and IBS, it rings true for me. I have found my body can get rapidly sensitized to various food groups.

*Your body–mind*
*is interlinked.*

So, let's just take it a little wider. In his ground-breaking book *When the Body Says No*, psychologist Gabor Maté explores the hidden cost of stress on the body. Maté suggests many health conditions are linked to childhood trauma and repressed emotion acting in the mind and body to cause a state of *dis*-ease. He also explores the findings of Dr Douglas Drossman, internationally known gastroenterologist and professor of medicine and psychiatry at the University of North Carolina, who suggested based on extensive clinical experience that there are psychosocial aspects to intestinal disease, and that chronically stressful emotional patterns may induce inflammatory disease in the gut.[13]

Well, I don't know about you, but when I read that, I felt some of that really chimes with me. For me, back at the start of my IBD journey, I didn't know anything about a gut diet or mental health. I thought I was just one of life's worriers. But I was struggling – and I was struggling to speak about it.

It's because chronic illnesses like ulcerative colitis, Crohn's disease and IBS are invisible that there is a real and present danger that we fail to express what's going on. We can be tempted to try and hold it all together. I did. There's a certain inner psychology to living with a chronic health condition. The actual process of getting your head around what your condition means for you. That, my dear, can take a bit of time.

## Shining the light on shame

Recently I rewatched Brené Brown's ground-breaking TED Talk on shame and thought, *to hell with it* (I think I'm channelling a little Texan when I say that), *I've got to tell this part of my story* – because living with chronic health conditions like IBD and IBS can feel shameful. Because the anxious gut is something that makes us play small and act with fear. We get anxious about the most mundane things. Eating out. Travelling. Visiting a friend. We start to preplan. Parties, concerts, festivals – all the fun stuff starts to exist against a background hum of anxiety. The many times I've apologized for not eating something that someone made or bought for me. IBD and IBS are invisible, and there's something about being hidden that can so easily slide into shame.

*Shine a light on shame, name it,*
*and you start to feel lighter.*

You can start to call it out gently, lovingly, firstly to yourself. So, how do you do that?

Well, for me, it was all about connecting to my gut in a whole new way – a tender, clear-sighted way. Looking shame in the eye and taking a deep belly breath and speaking to it with compassion and understanding. Making peace with fear and vulnerability because shame and fear ***feed*** our anxious gut.

The following practices are designed to open up a deeper, more authentic connection with your gut. My gut tells me that gut trouble is often fed by repressed emotion. So here you can give your gut more space to speak. Journalling can be a powerful tool to explore what's happening in your body, especially the energy that gets stuck in those dark corners of the ileum and colon. So, take out your Gut-loving Journal and have it ready.

## Learning gut compassion

When you know that stress has contributed to a flare, ask yourself the questions below in a loving, mindful way.

1. Find a comfortable position to lie down. I suggest bending your knees and placing your feet flat on the floor to enable your spine to lie flat. Close your eyes and come back to your deep base belly breathing (*see page 31* for a reminder) and renew that deep connection with your gut.

2. Once you have completed seven deep rounds of breathing, rest both of your palms gently on your belly area. Placing your hands on your belly can deepen the meditation. Now you can ask questions – saying the words slowly out loud to yourself:

    - For ulcerative colitis: 'My lovely colon, how can I help heal you?'
    - For Crohn's disease: 'My dear ileum, what is it I need to know?'
    - For IBS: 'My beautiful, bloated belly, what can I do to support you?'

3. After the question, take a few moments and give your gut wisdom time to respond. If you are experiencing a flare, you'll need to be especially gentle and spacious with your pain:

    - 'Hello, my tender inflammation, what is it that I need to know to heal?'
    - 'Hello, my dear pain, what is it that you wish to tell me?'
    - 'Dear anxiety, here we are again. How can I comfort you?'

4. Return back to deep base belly breathing, and you may find that images or words arise. I'm a visual person, so images and colours pop up for me. Depending on your own preference, you may experience sounds or sensations. As you start to tune in to your gut instinct, you may even start to hear a calm, clear voice of your gut wisdom emerge. The most important thing is to give your guts

loving space and the opportunity to be heard. The first time you try this, you may even draw a blank – that's OK too.

5. To close this practice, rest in your deepened base belly breathing and imagine healing light spreading through your fingers into your belly, cooling and healing the sites of inflammation or soothing places of bloating and pain.
6. Thank each part of your digestive tract for the wonderful job it's doing, and slowly open your eyes. This practice is particularly good to do in bed before going to sleep. You may even find your dreams will communicate further images or words to you.

When you start to listen deeply, you may discover that you've been setting off gut forest fires for years. This sad deforestation of your microbiome leaves patches of your villi barren and burned. You may have visions showing how your beautiful plicae circulares have been made raw from too much processed food. If you find that this is the case, it is important not to beat yourself up. Be gentle with yourself. This is a process.

*We start where we are right now.*

When you practise being present with all your emotions, you can show up for your whole self. Your anxious, churned-up gut needs to be acknowledged. When you give feelings and thoughts SPACE by simply breathing deeply and feeling them, naming them softly and journalling, you can start to acknowledge the whole gorgeous complex catastrophe of your being.

Let's go a little deeper into gut compassion. Remember, you are not trying to FIX your emotions. You cannot Marie Kondo your rage, your sadness, your shame. Emotions are energy, fluid and changeable.

## Anxious gut reflection

The following practice is particularly helpful if you're experiencing a flutter of anxiety or other strong emotions in your gut. To deepen this practice, I recommend completing it in nature if you can find a quiet, private place and ideally combine with bare feet on grass or earth.

1. Start the reflection process by grounding in your base belly practice. Take three breaths, and as you exhale, sigh outwardly as though you are misting a mirror. Now take your breath deeper down into your root chakra (*see figure 4, page 30*).

2. Turn your focused attention to the fluttering anxiety, pain or discomfort in your gut. Breathe into the sensation and exhale. Do this for a few minutes and until you start to feel the energy sitting behind the anxiety and discomfort. You may notice a buzzing warmth. You may even notice as you focus on the feeling that it increases; that's totally natural. Don't try to do anything. Just keep breathing gently, lovingly into the sensation.

3. As you keep breathing into the anxiety or pain, you may notice it start to shift and move. Observe that. Often, we treat our 'negative' feelings by pushing against them, and for those of us with gut trouble, we can literally swallow them down. You know how our language reveals the *gut-wrenching* and *gut-twisting* emotions we hold here.

4. As you feel the emotion, say their names softly like you might whisper to an old friend (who is just trying to help you out): anxiety, shame, sadness, fear, frustration. Whatever feelings arise, gently acknowledge them. If you are standing on the earth, you may feel a sense of earthing and calming naturally arise.[14]

5. Giving our unexpressed emotions a gentle space naturally starts to soften, then to loosen those stuck patterns of energy that have been hanging around for a while. The breath has a kind of soothing magic, it can act to calm the gut–brain axis, and crucially as we breathe with awareness, it can help us be present with and ***process*** our emotions.

6. To close the exercise, exhale out the worry, anxiety, pain. Finish when you feel a lighter, more energized feeling. If you feel that there is still much to work through, trust that the simple act of giving these feelings space is the start of healing.

7. Take a few moments to journal.

This is a particularly powerful practice to do in the morning. If you still feel that you have deep unfinished work, which you may, please invest time to go deeper. Healing happens in our heart, gut and head. As we heal, we start to align all these parts of ourselves. You may wish to seek out support from a counsellor or coach. See Resources at the end for ideas on reading.

If you want to see a brave face in transforming shame, take a look at the irrepressible joy of @lottiedrynan on Instagram. Lottie went from obsessive dieting to bloat love, and she shares her story (The Tummy Diaries) with a smile.

# CHAPTER 6

# THE COMPASSIONATE GUT

*'When you are compassionate with yourself, you trust in your soul, which you let guide your life. Your soul knows the geography of your destiny better than you do.'*

JOHN O' DONOHUE, IRISH POET,
*ANAM CARA: A BOOK OF CELTIC WISDOM*

A compassionate commitment to gut wellbeing will help heal your gut. We know greater self-compassion lowers levels of inflammation in the body. But greater self-compassion is also about how you show up in life for yourself.

We know that our personal food map is important in shaping our gut health, and creating a healthy, individualized gut-led diet is crucial to reducing irritability and inflammation. But let's face it, many of us already have a pretty unhealthy relationship with the 'F word': fad diets, eating disorders, the restrictions of 'clean eating' offering the promise of a new you. Those of us living with IBD and IBS have an extra layer of 'food fear', making us easy prey for diets that promise a lot if we follow their complex restrictions.

There's a real risk of developing orthorexia – an eating disorder caused by hyper anxiety about what we can and can't eat. This is not the spirit of this book. My mission is to support you in discovering your best gut health. An elimination diet can be a crucial ally on the road to good gut health, but we need to start from a freeing mindset with gut compassion and self-compassion at its foundation.

As you read this section, make your commitment to whatever you decide to do from a deeply grounded place of loving your whole gut. The psychology of self-care is a core part of the healing journey, so let's have a look at one of the key areas that might derail the process before you even begin to make changes.

## Dealing with 'f**k it, one piece won't kill me'

This is an important issue for sticking to an elimination diet and then successfully avoiding trigger foods. What I have learned about sustaining clear changes to my food intake is that it's helpful to get really clear on your **motivation**. When 'f**k it, I'll have a slice of cake, a swig of beer' arises, what's your driver to not go there, right at that moment?

The answer is about building a clear-sighted foundation through gut knowledge towards gut compassion and gut healing. When I look at my food porn – fresh, hot, soft, wheat pizza – and I want a slice, I think of my beloved colon, which I thank each and every day, and my brain.

As we extend our gut knowledge and deepen our gut compassion, we understand that inflammation – especially ongoing inflammation – takes a toll not just on the gut but on many different areas of the body, including the heart and brain. The lens of self-compassion allows us to see our gut health in a wider body context. It helps us connect the dots of our gut knowledge in a whole new way.

One recent large-scale study involving 250,000 people with IBD revealed that those of us living with elevated levels of inflammation have twice the risk of heart attacks long term than those living without IBD.[15] Another study of neuroinflammation (inflammation on brain function) is starting to shine a light on how systemic inflammation contributes to conditions like Parkinson's disease and dementia.[16] Not only does inflammation increase the likelihood of low mood and depression, but it can also play a role in a wide range of illnesses. So those are the facts, and too easily they may drive change through fear, and well, to quote from Yoda: 'Fear leads to anger. Anger leads to hate. Hate leads to suffering.' To make long-term, sustained changes, we must find the deeper motivation beyond our fear and self-judgement and instead act from a deep sense of self-care.

## Grow your fierce self-compassion

Find what you are motivated by – the stronger the emotion, the better. That emotion will help you cut through the 'f**k it' thinking pretty quickly. The short exercise detailed below will help you clarify your motivation.

What's your motivation? Your waistline, your skin, just the sheer hellish boredom of being in bloated pain – again. You know that once you fall off that particular *fear-motivated bandwagon* (and you will, sooner or later), you just start to beat yourself up all over again. It's just at that point you're easy prey to 'f**k it' thinking. You'll be tempted to eat all the foods that cause you harm. And, well, we know just how easy that is to do because it's the food that pretty much everybody else is eating.

So instead, you'll need a good grounding in fierce self-compassion. You'll need to be so tuned in to your deeper self-care needs that you can navigate through the superficial pull to do all the wrong stuff with ease.

To make changes to your diet as part of a sustained gut-healing, anti-inflammatory lifestyle, you need to be fully grounded in a clear-sighted ***internal gut-led*** motivation grounded in self-compassion. So, as you begin to understand the wider interplay between your gut health and inflammatory lifestyle triggers – pollutants, poor sleep, low levels of exercise, diet, food allergies and stress – you'll start to feel empowered to do the right thing by your gut.

## Your f**k it motivation maker

Take a deep, fiercely compassionate breath, get your Gut-loving Journal and reflect on the following questions:

- What is your deepest **driver towards** the health and life you want? If you're not sure, then start with what you find hardest about living with a chronic illness. What's your deepest health fear? Yes, the one you've never told anyone about. Put it down here for a moment – a picture, words, a few lines. OK, that's powerful motivation; a **'driver away from'**. Good to clarify and often helpful in the short term. But it's not enough for long-term sustained change.
- So let's flip this back to your **driver towards**, what do you want to move towards? What's the best vision you have for a healthy gut and a healthy life? Write that down. Better still, create an image.

You matter. Your wellbeing matters. The quality of your life matters. And you can do this. Trust that your actions have the power to move you forwards into healing. What's really interesting about this exercise is that it focuses your mind on what you think matters because it's the driver of your actions. External reasons for change and fear don't tend to stick long term. The data, the big facts, have a way of washing over us. So it's time to trust the wisdom and wonder of your microbiome and trust that you can make a change.

*Compassion naturally flows as self-awareness of gut wellbeing grows.*

## Belly Metta Bhavana practice

The following practices are designed to shine a light on your hidden gut organs. To give them a voice, so they become real places in your inner body that deserve to be treated with mindful attention. *Maitrī* or *Mettā* are found in Vedic Sanskrit texts (the root word derives from 'mid', which translates simply as 'love'). This ancient practice will support you in stretching and developing your self-love muscle, and once this is strengthened, you'll find this naturally expands outwards into the rest of your life.

The Metta Bhavana meditation from the Theravada Buddhist tradition begins with directing loving-kindness towards yourself. This is the foundation of all compassion practices: to love outwardly, we must first love inwardly. In this case, to truly love ourselves, we must honour and love our inner organs – your dear gut. The following practice is a simple daily loving-kindness takeaway. Once you have committed to the deeper work of somatically processing your emotions and experiencing and expressing your feelings (*see practice on page 73*), you can use this simple practice to keep connecting in a loving, healing way to your gut.

### Belly Metta Bhavana practice

The Metta Bhavana practice is a rich and ancient kindness mantra for developing loving-kindness and cultivating greater self-compassion. The heart of the traditional practice is the refrain: 'May I be well, may I be happy, may I be safe.'

1. To start, close your eyes and return to your base belly breath (*see page 31*). Again, placing your palms on your belly to enrich the focus and depth of the practice.

2. When you feel ready, lightly and gently focus on your Belly Metta Bhavana mantra. Choose the words and images that feel right to heal yourself and arise for you during this exercise. I've suggested some simple ones but be creative and use what resonates with you.

   - May my belly be well, may it be healed, may it be safe.
   - May my belly be gently nourished by this meal.
   - May my bloated belly be soothed. May it be blessed.
   - May my colon [*ileum or any part of your gut*] be calm, may my colon be healed, may my colon be whole.
   - May I feel peace, may I feel strong, may I feel whole.
   - May I learn to love and listen to my gut.

3. Repeat your chosen mantra softly to yourself until you feel a sense of the words filling your body and your belly.

4. When you are ready, gently open your eyes and move back into your day, carrying the soothing words of your mantra with you.

5. Continue to repeat your chosen mantra softly under your breath or even out loud throughout your day. Let the words bring you back to your breath and your belly over and over.

---

The traditional Metta Bhavana focuses on developing self-care and compassion and then moving this loved-up compassion outwards. First, towards somebody you love, then to somebody you feel neutral about. Then outwards towards somebody you have difficulty with, and ultimately towards all beings everywhere. By strengthening your self-compassion muscle, you become more loving in how you show up to yourself and others!

## The benefits of kindness

In *The Five Side Effects of Kindness*,[17] David Hamilton shares the benefits of kindness. There's a lot of science to show that kindness is good for us and the path of true change. When we are ill, we have a deep need for kindness. Our energetic imprints are particularly powerful for people who are ill. Never underestimate the need for kindness and gentle, compassionate care for anyone who is seriously ill or at the end of their life.

In my own stay in the hospital, I felt stripped of the external energetic layer: the etheric field. The etheric field is a thin invisible shield of protective energy which encloses the healthy body during wellness, but gets eroded when we are seriously ill. This field's fragmentation can heighten our sensitivity towards others' emotional and energetic vibrations. This leaves us feeling vulnerable and more sensitized, and therefore it is also an opportunity to tune in to our deeper gut-led longings.

As your gut compassion starts to calm your bloated belly and anxious mind, you'll start to feel more connected. As though your heart, head and gut are in alignment. And then the magic happens. You'll naturally feel more motivated to follow through on those things you know are gut healing – your goals. In this way, compassion becomes the bridge between your growing gut knowledge and your actions, easing the path to healing. You'll also start to notice that the small voice within grows louder as the pull of your intuition naturally nudges you in different situations. As you become more attuned to your deeper gut instincts, you'll naturally be more mindful of your choices.

CHAPTER 7

# THE MINDFUL FOOD FLOW

*'Let your curiosity be greater than your fear.'*

PEMA CHÖDRÖN, BUDDHIST TEACHER AND AUTHOR

Animals in their natural environment are deeply attuned to their bodies' needs. Heeding these subtle messages, they seek out food even at great risk to themselves. A mountain goat will climb a vertical dam to eat calcium residue. Wild and domestic animals eat charcoal, obeying an instinct to detoxify their digestive system. In Borneo, researchers have spotted orangutans selecting handfuls of iron-rich soil around their nests to supplement their plant-based diet.

### ♥ Gut Love ♥

Boost your gut-loving friendly fibre today to nourish your beautiful Bifidobacteria and lovely lactobacillus by eating fermented foods like kefir and sauerkraut, and eating whole oats.

We urban humans – sitting long hours in temperature-controlled rooms – are so often disconnected from our natural instincts. In the average Western diet, there is an easy tendency to eat a limited range of highly processed foods. The beige heavyweights of wheat, dairy, sugar and processed fats are the staple ingredients in ready meals and fast food.

Something that's not often discussed is how sustaining a different diet from the 'norm' takes courage. The easy options, the stuff the average UK person eats in the 2020s, are generally gut limiting. Eating fresh, whole food takes dedication, consistency and a fair slice of gut knowledge and gut compassion.

## The mindful food flow principle – nurturing healthy gut instinct

For my part, after leaving hospital, I continued to nurture my growing sense of self-compassion. To my surprise, this self-compassion awoke my gut instincts. My body started to feel a new, deep, gut-level connection to food. As my body healed, it would wake me in the night with **food longings.** I would creep into the kitchen and find myself drawn to just what felt like the 'right' foods: avocados, carrots, extra virgin olive oil.

It was in that space of slow recovery that my long-lost instincts awoke. I would hold food in my hands – skin to gnarly root flesh – for a few seconds and feel a lightness, a rising longing in my gut. The first time I used this technique, shortly after I left hospital, I was significantly underweight with a body mass index (BMI) of 16. I struggled to eat large meals and found my body became a dowsing rod to the food it needed.

### ♥ Gut Love ♥

There is evidence that butyric acid, found in foods like extra virgin olive oil, heals the lining of the gut.

Even today, whenever I feel those first flickerings of *itis*, I slow down and re-engage with my gut. I choose to shop in the quiet, early morning. I take some deep base belly breaths, and as I walk the aisles of the fresh food counters of the market or health-food store, I connect with my gut.

Sometimes when passing through the veg section in my local supermarket, I've found myself drawn to pineapple – it contains bromelain, a protein-digesting enzyme with anti-inflammatory properties, so good for gorgeous guts. This is why it's best to avoid shopping when hungry or when the market is busy, as it blurs the intuitive pull of food.

The following exercise will help you start to tune in to your food, but a word of warning: you can be subject to false positives due to the superficial pull that most mammals have to sugar and fat – the unhealthy kinds. On finding a ripe fruit tree, our ancestral relatives, the hunter-gatherers, would gorge themselves on the rare, glucose-rich, easy-energy fuel – think chancing upon a honey hive or mango tree. We've got thousands of years of evolution pushing us to do just that. These same habits still apply today, but now glucose-rich food is readily available. This has now become a dangerous instinct, which explains the obesity and diabetes epidemics of the West. On the other hand, the compassionate gut pull has a different quality – a subtler, wholesome, healing sensation. Distinguishing the compassionate pull from the superficial may take a little practice and refinement.

When we relearn ways to choose and prepare food with love and respect – for ourselves and the ingredients – we recognize that what we eat travels a long distance through our inner world. Depending on your digestive transit time, the ingredients will travel with us for 24–72 hours. Each day we use nutrients to repair and rebuild our bodies, so our food is with us for much longer than that.

The more you learn to follow your deeper gut instinct, the more you can literally touch food and feel an energetic pull to eat it. If you start to really see and feel the organs of your gut as an integral part of you, as worthy of your compassion, you can then start to love them back to health.

## Intuitive eating guide

This intuitive eating exercise is a great way of honing your instincts and learning to trust your gut. Try it for the first time at home in the kitchen before trying it out at the supermarket or health store.

1. Start by taking a few mindful base belly breaths and turn inwards to tune in to your deep gut intuition.
2. Hold the food in your hand and take a few moments to find the full sensory connection with this food. I find that if I close my eyes, I have a more powerful connection with my gut instinct. If you can, unwrap it from any packaging and hold it to you, skin to skin, but equally it can work in a container. Hold it to your nose and inhale deeply.
3. At this stage, you may feel really ***drawn*** to the food, feel a real sense of connection and even longing. Or you may feel aversion, subtle or strong. Attune to that feeling. It may be around your stomach area, or it may also be much more delicate, barely noticeable. Sometimes I can feel a subtle irritation – a muddy, sticky feeling arises, and I know that food isn't right for me.
4. Take a few moments to meditate on this sensation. Remember, if you consume this food, it will travel 9m (29ft 6in) along your gorgeous digestive tract.
5. I have learned over time the food that 'speaks my language' – the food that will heal my gut lining and care for my microbiome. Go gently and smile to your gut lovelies as you do this practice.

When your body really, intuitively wants a food, it's a different, deeper/lighter feeling than a desire for Dunkin' Donuts. Be receptive, keep practising intuitive eating, and you will find your responses will become more attuned and powerful. You may even find you feel differently as the seasons change. Our bodies have different needs across the year: warming foods are essential in the autumn and winter months, and cooler, raw foods are more natural for our bodies to digest in the late spring and summer. Go slowly as you do this, and you'll also train your microbiome and create a cycle of greater gut integrity and gut healing.

Ironically, at times of stress or anxiety, we are often drawn to the very foods that cause the greatest difficulty to our dear digestive tract, triggering a mix of inflammatory and autoimmune responses which can create a vicious spiral. At times when we are already placing a strain on our system with overwork or lack of sleep, these poor food choices can complete the destructive cycle for our gut. Practise rediscovering your gut instincts, and that still small voice will start to strengthen. Your intuition will flourish. Treat it like a well-loved plant: tend to it, hear it and it will serve you well. You will start to feel lighter, more whole.

## No grain, no pain

Trusting your gut instinct may require you to remove a specific food from your personal food map. For me, wheat is an inflammatory agent, and some highly processed forms are particular triggers. Stodgy Chorleywood processed bread – on the surface light and fluffy but pinch a small piece and roll it between finger and thumb, and it forms a hard moist lump. Just imagine what it does to the delicate lining of your villi. Another protein called amylase-trypsin inhibitors (ATIs) (found in wheat, barley and rye) has been shown to cause strong immune reactions in some people. There is even evidence of it being linked to IBD.[18] So if in doubt, leave the gluten out and bake your own gluten-free sourdough or soda bread.

But why is wheat such a problem?

In part, there's been an over-reliance on this little, plump grain of goodness for a long time – pizza, pasta, pastries, cereals and, of course, BREAD. I don't know about you – but I love it. But before jumping on the gluten-free wagon, let's take a brief look at why gluten may be emerging as such a villain!

Somewhere in the late 1960s, the bread industry lost the plot. Supermarkets needed quick, easy mass-produced loaves that travelled. The Chorleywood baking method sped up the baking process, making it cheaper and enabling the use of lower-quality, low-protein wheat. Bread moved from small-scale local bakeries to a billion-dollar industry. Bread needed to stay fresh and fluffy in a nice, plastic package (yeah, plastic, well that's a whole other story) for as long as possible and, hey presto, the sliced white loaf was born. Today around 80 per cent of UK bread makers use this method, and the bread is shipped worldwide.[19] This type of fast-baked loaf needs around two to three times the yeast of traditionally baked bread – feeling a little gassy, anyone?

To make this bread travel- and shelf-fresh, it has a few extras thrown in: enzymes, preservatives and a few antifungals – just to make sure this spongy, high-water-content bread doesn't go mouldy.

In fact, there is growing evidence of a condition called non-coeliac gluten sensitivity (NCGS). In this condition, the immune system overreacts to the presence of gluten. There's also been some speculation whether this is due to the bread-making process and the addition of enzymes and increased yeast or trace fertilizers and chemicals in the wheat grain. The NCGS condition may in part explain the spread of our modern bloated bellies.

And while it's inspiring to see a generation push back with varied grains, and homemade and artisan sourdough, it's clear too many of us are eating highly industrialized grains which are doing us and our guts no good.

### *Industrialized gut*

We know that our food habits can turn us into food addicts. Our industrialized guts are co-evolving with the foods we eat. Processed foods need a shelf life. Preservatives and emulsifiers are excellent chemical concoctions for helping foods last longer, but they're less good for the delicate balance of our gut microbiome. These non-food additives are a little like food detergents. And well, they're no good for our gut.

Our food choices are big business – the scale of specialized production in Western culture is immense as 50 per cent of the world's plant-based carbohydrates come from three crops: wheat, corn and rice.

Manufactured food is leaving its mark on our inner ecosystem. It's starting to shape the microbiome of much wider global communities in countries with a diverse, non-Western diet. This is partly due to how a small group of grains are now global key players and partly due to the widespread use of antibiotics – particularly in pregnancy.

You may have even found in your own gut story (*see page 37*) that the use of antibiotics when your mum was pregnant or in the early part of your life played a factor in your own gut troubles. We know from research that 'antibiotics change the baby's inherited microbial communities with long-term disease consequences'.[20] Of course, there is no one microbiome – we are each unique – but there is evidence of an imbalanced biome in the unhealthy gut. The good news – you get to shape the profile of your inner landscape.

## What you eat can help or hinder

It takes time and practice to break the habits of 'easy eating'. Interestingly, if you practice mindful shopping and eating (*see page 86*), you may find foods on the free-from shelves are not always right for you. They may not be the stuff to feed your beautiful microbiome and nurture your gut. Every time you eat, try to breathe, tune in to your belly and 'feel' if it's the right thing. The right food will create a lightness, a feeling of connection and 'fit' as though the food is resonating at an energetic healing level.

So the big news is to **follow your gut**. In doing this, you will start to develop gut integrity and quite literally learn to follow what makes you feel good when you eat, while you eat and very much afterwards. If you are always bloated, uneasy and uncomfortable after eating, however much you (and some of those inner gut bugs) may love that food, face it, it's not for you.

## Being present with your plate

Most of us are pretty clear that *what we eat* is significant to our gut health. What's sometimes startled me is that the *way we eat* can be just as important. Mindless eating is the norm. Blink and you miss it, and half of us regularly eat our meal in front of the TV.[21] Well, let's drop the judgement but just acknowledge this is not good for us or our gut bugs.

There's a science to this process. When we slow down and breathe deeply, we increase blood flow to our gut. When we eat slowly and chew our food thoroughly, not only do we start the mechanical part of digestion (*see page 6*), but we also stimulate the salivary glands and the enzyme amylase.

So the *way* you approach eating shapes how your digestive system responds. If like me, you are one of life's rapid eaters, then you have probably spent a lifetime swallowing food quickly and mindlessly. In times of stress, speed eating is the norm. Let's suspend judgement. Have you ever noticed just how much our culture worships at the altar of speed? Urgency is a badge of honour in the workplace – getting the job done. And that tendency can spill over into our eating: on-the-run breakfasts, lunches crouched over laptops, rapid-fire dinners.

One secret to removing habits that no longer serve you is to create simple, new rituals. These act like hooks to help embed change.

## The simple hook of grace

Grace is all about smoothness or elegance of movement – a gift to your gut. Of course, there's a deeper resonance to grace, a more spiritual meaning. Grace implies stillness, and if you still have a tendency towards mindless mechanical fuelling to the theme tune of your favourite Netflix series, then you are not enabling a relationship of grace with your plate. Grace sets the tone of a meal, creating a little ceremony to mark the point where you take a moment, even a micro-moment, to slow down. And as you slow, you can bring presence to your plate and mindful compassion to your gut.

So how can we be more present?

Whilst cooking, list the ingredients to get more attuned to food diversity – we're going to explore just how important that is in Part III. Feel gratitude to the makers, bakers, farmers, pickers, packagers and transporters. On an average day, I sprinkle Indonesian cinnamon on my morning porridge, crush French garlic into the dressing of Portuguese salad leaves, grind a little Keralan black pepper on my tofu and pluck an Ecuadorian banana for a mid-afternoon snack.

How about you?

In even a micro-moment of grace, you might want to reflect on that web of folk linked to your plate. You've probably heard of the theory of 'six degrees of separation'? It turns out it's true – well, it averages at 6.6 measures of social separation between any two people on Earth – meaning it's possible to trace our relationship with any person on the planet in under seven different connections. Apply this to food and wow – the sheer number of folk who make a meal possible is startling. The food on our plate holds history and interconnection.

Family mealtimes and weekends are a great chance to slow into grace. Once established, you can use a shorter micro gut-grace. Keep it fresh – and if you have kids, let them lead. It's a chance for a deep dive into the sources of your food. Be radical. Offer to say grace if you're sharing a meal with friends or colleagues.

## Gut grace

### Being present with your plate

Appreciating the content and context of your plate is an act of gut care. I want to share grace with you because the most powerful thing about sharing grace is the act of honouring your gut.

1. Grace is gratitude. Take a deep breath, and as you exhale, look at your plate. Let the food be your inspiration.

2. Grace is like a musical refrain. The themes are gratitude and celebration. Name each food briefly and visualize its journey to your plate. Thank each person in the food chain who nurtured and carried this food to you. Think of their hands.

3. Reflect on the food's final journey through your 9m (29ft 6in) long digestive tract. The phytonutrients, amino acids and vitamins form the building blocks of cells. Thank your food, ask it to heal your beloved gut, and nourish your dear gut bugs.

4. Wrap grace around your meal. When you have finished, place your hands lovingly on your belly and trust your gut to do the inner work.

In a culture that celebrates speed over slowness, **it's up to us to reclaim our calm**. We speed up, we notice, so we slow down because sustained change requires fierce and loving self-compassion. We're talking about a self-care revolution. To change the environment of your life is a significant act. You start where you are.

CHAPTER 8

# SLEEP CARE IS GUT CARE

*'Sleep that knits up the ravelled sleave of care, Balm of hurt minds, ...Chief nourisher in life's feast.'*

WILLIAM SHAKESPEARE, *MACBETH*

Sleep heals. It's that simple. When we sleep, the body gets the chance to rest and reset. When we don't get sufficient sleep, we can fall prey to a whole host of physical and mental health issues. The sad reality is that we are living in increasingly sleepless cities.[22] Poor sleep almost certainly plays a key role in anxiety and stress. Studies show that as little as two days of too little sleep can increase cortisol levels and inflammation, subtly impacting our gut bugs' balance.[23]

**Gut Love**

Late at night, your beloved bowels are busy working hard. Breathe deeply into your own gut dance.

In fact, fatigue and obesity often go hand in hand. Lack of sleep causes us to seek out sources of energy – sugar and fat. We are pulled to the very inflammatory foods, which feed the less healthy bacteria in our microbiome. This can create a negative cycle, unsettling our microbiome and increasing inflammation, making us feel tired and unwell. So protecting your sleep is part and parcel of protecting your gut wellbeing.[24]

## Reclaiming your sleep

OK, let's start with the simplest practical steps to sorting sleep. Make reclaiming your bedroom an act of JOY. Protect your environment because the space you sleep in is precious, so get Gut Shui-ing.

### ♥ Gut Love ♥

The purpose of your bedroom is to sleep and have sex, so if you struggle with sleep, take a look at the space you offer yourself each night-time and honestly ask yourself, is it fit for purpose? Take a look right now. Would you offer this space to a dear friend, right now, as it is? If not, why not?

### *Tips for good Gut Shui and sleep hygiene*

- Invest in a mattress that makes you want to sink into its embrace. An inexpensive way to do this is to get an excellent quality mattress topper.
- Turn the radiator settings to low – a cool room aids sleep.
- Choose simplicity and soft tones. Colours create wavelengths of light that increase or decrease heart rate. Choose a colour scheme of pale blues, whites or soft greens.[25]

- Declutter with fierce, focused compassion. Your bedroom is not the place for the laundry basket, kids' toys or overspill from your home office.

- Sleep needs darkness, but our light-saturated cityscapes hide the stars and bleed through the curtains and blinds.[26] Invest in blackout blinds and curtains that will make your room dark. This is particularly important in summer as this sensitivity to light is embedded in our biology. We have photoreceptors in our bodies that impact our hormones.

- Choose natural anti-inflammatory materials for your bedding and nightclothes (if you wear them) – 100 per cent cotton, silk or bamboo. Add fragrance with organic oils and scents rather than artificial air-fresheners and plugs-in (it's important to protect our biome and reduce the chemical footprint of our home environment; natural oils also have a physiological impact on hormones). Include plants that oxygenate and purify the air – aloe vera, peace lilies or gerbera daisies.

## Seven steps towards gut-soothing sleep

OK, so now you've sorted out your space, it's time to compassionately create some new loving sleep rituals. A little ceremony can help to create new healthy habits to support a more mindful life, which will lead to better sleep. But let's keep it light, nothing too heavy or too ritualistic. You don't want to replace one set of anxieties with another. First, just admit how many things are encroaching on the edges of your sleep and then lean towards incorporating the following seven steps to upgrade your sleep:

### *1. What to eat for sleep*

A healthy microbiome helps us sleep, and there's a whole field of study opening up around this. People with healthy, diverse microbiomes with high levels of phylum Bacteroidetes have deeper, more efficient sleep.[27] Foods high in fibre and rich in protein promote a higher quality of sleep.[28] So think probiotics, such as lactobacillus and bifidobacteria for an anti-anxiety effect'.[29]

Prebiotic-rich foods like garlic, artichoke and onions can help to improve sleep and support your gut microbiota. Even more fascinating is how what we eat might impact not just the amount of sleep we get, but the quality too. Recent studies in animals show that those on a prebiotic diet spent more time in restorative non-rapid-eye-movement (NREM) sleep. After stress, they also spent more time in rapid-eye-movement (REM) sleep, which is critical for recovery from stress.[30]

Avoid saturated fat, carbs and high-sugar foods, particularly before bedtime, as they can disrupt sleep by destabilizing blood sugar. So the good old anti-inflammatory lifestyle, Mediterranean or plant-based, helps sleep for a range of reasons by supporting a healthy microbiome, reducing anxiety levels and supporting the lowering of inflammation in the brain.

There are clear links between gut microbiome composition, sleep physiology, the immune system and cognition, which the new field of psychobiotics is starting to open up. The relationship between our gut and our brain is an exciting research area, so watch this space for more human-scale studies and what this will mean for gut-loving sleep. We'll explore how to feed the good bacteria in Part III.

**♥ Gut Love ♥**

Fermented foods feed your microbiome. Try kimchi, sauerkraut or homemade kombucha.

### *2. What to drink for sleep*

In winter, try a glass of warm tryptophan-rich almond milk with a grate of serotonin-rich, fresh nutmeg before bed. Mix it up in summer with chamomile or valerian tea. You have to time it right, so it doesn't lead you to a night-time toilet trip. Choose your best mug or cup on a beautiful saucer. To deepen the sense of ritual, light an oil burner (add a few drops of soothing lavender) and create this as a moment of tranquillity to mark the end of your day, a pivot point to sleep.

Avoid alcohol and caffeine, and energy drinks during the day. These are all sleep disruptors.

**♥ Gut Love ♥**

Have a cup of carminative mint tea after dinner. Mint is an easy-growing perennial. Pick a few sprigs and add to hot water, steep for a few minutes and enjoy a home-grown organic mint tea.

### *3. Drop the worry ball – simple rituals for calm*

We all know that sleep is important to our wellbeing, and there is a risk of creating a new level of sleep anxiety. So how do you turn sleep into your gut ally and friend?

**Journalling:** If you are always busy with an overactive mind, give yourself the gift of space. Spill out all those worries on to a pad either before or when you get into bed. Doodle, draw and rant your worries. Julia Cameron, the author of *The Artist's Way*,[31] advocates Morning Pages as a way of enabling the unconscious mind, which is so closely attuned to our deeper gut instincts, to have free rein in our lives.

**Worry jar:** One way to park worries directly before bedtime is to create a worry jar to store those incomplete to-do lists and stop them swirling around your head in the wee hours.

**Get acquainted:** I've been gently, humorously getting to know my inner insomniac. So now I know what helps her when she wakes at 3 a.m., believing she's got to send an email or plan a meal. I've been talking her down for a while, and now we're pretty close. We've got a relationship built on 'no bullshit' – just love. I have her back, and she knows it. If it's between her and work, she wins every time. Just knowing that seems to soothe her. Building a relationship with your good self, your gorgeous gut, is vital.

**Find a restful podcast:** I love the soothing voices of Elizabeth Gilbert and Pema Chödrön. Find yours, and you will have a night-time buddy and psychological solace.

## *4. Mindful movement for gut sleep*

Investing a bit of time in the day to reframe your psychological approach to your night-time habits is an act of self-care. The opposite of fear is not courage but compassion. So breathe and exhale... Sleep is an act of letting go, but when we are most stressed and anxious, it can feel almost impossible. We are wired up on cortisol and adrenaline, gulping back cups of coffee and high-sugar snacks.

If this sounds familiar, then re-establish your relationship with the process of letting go and letting be in your waking life. Simple mindfulness practices are wonderful opportunities to learn to let go. Literally learning to tune in to the natural calm of your parasympathetic nervous system. Go, vagus, you know what to do. And if, like me, you are genetically primed to wake up in the night, then create a night-time breath practice and get into yoga.

## Gut-loving yoga

### Cat/cow

It's possible to gently stimulate the vagus nerve with yoga postures that open your chest and throat. Do this stretch for you and your beloved gut. Keep them simple and slow and listen to your body. As you breathe, focus on your exhalation, allow yourself to expand into the open heart and soft belly of your gut. This lovely flowing movement (vinyasa) enables you to bring awareness to the rhythm of your breath.

1. Ensure you have a comfy blanket or yoga mat and move into a wide-armed/knee table position on all fours. Align your wrists with your shoulders and your knees with your hips.

2. Cow pose. As you inhale, curl your toes under, tilt your pelvis so that your tailbone sticks up. As you do this, begin to lift your head and your hips lowering your belly towards the floor into cow pose.

3. On your exhale, uncurl your toes, so your feet rest on the floor, tip your pelvis forward, letting your spine round into cat pose. Let your head drop, and as you do, gaze at your beautiful belly.

4. Find your own flow to this after around seven cycles, pause and take a deep belly breath and move to a neutral position and then slowly ease out of the posture. Follow the flow of your own breath and listen to your body.

### *5. Get perspective by starlight*

Spending time lying on the earth creates a sense of calm. In my second week in the hospital, I managed to find a patch of grass to lie down on. Although my cannula and nasogastric tube might have worried a few onlookers, I felt a deep level of earthy joy just getting out of the sterile hospital ward and into nature for an hour. Some studies have even shown that regular earthing has a health impact on the body.[32]

If you have a garden, get a rug and lie on the ground and watch the sky and the stars. When we are anxious and stressed, we feel the spotlight of the world is on us. There is something deeply grounding in resting on Mother Earth and feeling the solar system's vastness. No garden? Then gaze upwards out of a window, find a piece of the sky and breathe into the cool night air. Repeat. Combine with corpse pose for a deepening impact.

## Yoga to tune in to your rest-and-reset system

### Corpse pose

Yoga can calm the nervous system. For this exercise, you'll need a yoga mat or comfy rug. On a warm day, soft grass is perfect too

1. Find a quiet place (on the earth outside if possible). Lie down on the ground and nestle into a flat-backed extended position; adjust, so you feel fully held by the earth beneath you.

2. Let your hands flop to your sides, palms upwards. Let your legs naturally part in a way that releases any tension in your lower back. Your feet may flop to the sides.

3. Start to notice your breath. Let your face, jaw and muscles fully relax.

4. Complete a gentle check-in with your body, focusing on each body part in turn. As you do this, combine deep, slow, natural breaths.

5. Let your exhale be effortless. If you feel any tension, bring your awareness to this and breathe gently into it and watch it slowly dissolve. Trust and rest.

6. Do this as long as you feel you need to – and you will have a deeper, more restful sleep.

7. When you exit from this position, do it gently (with eyes closed), bring your knees slowly to your chest and then roll to one side, and rest there for a few breaths. Move slowly up to a sitting position and then to bed.

For more yoga poses, see *page 167*.

## *6. Love thy belly massage*

I bake bread each Sunday morning, and it fills the house with a wholesome, warming homey-ness. Smell directly impacts the nervous system; scent molecules hit the olfactory nerves and head to our amazing amygdala, the almond-shaped emotional centre of the brain. Aromatherapy aids relaxation, improves sleep, relieves anxiety and depression, and improves perceived life quality for those with chronic health conditions.

If you feel bloated and in general digestive distress, a gentle belly massage is a lovely evening ritual – a hook for a new habit. So this evening, put down your phone/tablet and invest in some gut-loving care.

Avoid massaging straight after a large meal. Let your gut settle and do its wonder work before applying any pressure. Think about the beautiful three-sided large intestine around the central folded concertinaed small intestine (*see figure 2, page 6*). This is the frame of your massage.

If you have a partner, ask them to massage your belly and guide them on the pressure. You don't want to add top-down pressure to your organs. Having someone else gently massaging your abdominal area is profoundly gut relaxing. It's the exact opposite of gut-wrenching. So if you have had a particularly stressful and gut-twisting day, building in a gentle belly rub-down is an act of pure gut love. You deserve it.

Go gently with the tender belly of your body. In the natural world, animals turn over and expose their delicate underbelly as an act of surrender. So choose your massage partner wisely. Be confident to state if the pressure gets too heavy. If you are in severe discomfort and during a flare, don't add pressure. Instead lie down, take a small amount of oil, inhale and hold your belly gently, and toggle your hands to your breath and to your belly to synchronize your breathing as we have done in the base belly breathing exercise.

## ♥ Gut Love ♥

Feeling tense? Try this anytime: in a seated position, place your hands palm upwards on your knees and as you breathe in slowly, softly close your fists. As you exhale, release your hands to a soft open position. Do this for a count of seven. Your breathing will naturally start to slow.

### *Creating your own personal gut-love massage oil blend*

Almond or coconut oil makes an ideal base blend massage oil. At night, a small amount of warmed coconut oil mixed with a few drops of your favourite oil blend can create a soothing and moisturising massage oil. (Bonus: it also can be gorgeous mixed into your hair as an extra deep-conditioning treatment.) Almond oil is a more neutral blend oil, but you can also use flaxseed or juniper. Warm the mixture in your hands and keep it warm so that it is spreadable.

For stress and overwhelm during the daytime, eucalyptus is an antispasmodic oil that can refresh your mind and bring clarity.

Yarrow was used traditionally to reduce abdominal pain and inflammation.[33] A few drops of anti-inflammatory rosemary[34] in your favourite carrier oil can also ease bloating. Peppermint oil is a great all-rounder for IBS relief,[35] while clove is a special spice packed with polyphenols – it stimulates metabolism and is an anti-inflammatory.

For an evening belly massage, a good all-around oil like lavender is an ideal blend. If you're new to aromatherapy, it is a simple, safe starter oil with calming and pain-relieving properties. It's the one you'll have heard about for getting a better night's sleep.

Ideally, try and go for a base, mid and top-note mix of oils. This works to create a complementary blend. But once you have got the basics, play with the smells and create your own unique blend. You might even want to mix up a batch and give it a name: Gut love flare mix.

If you want to explore a little deeper, oils like Roman chamomile and vetiver have been shown to boost the immune system. Frankincense is a warming sedative oil that can create a sense of peace and comfort. I use it during my evening meditation practice.

*Note:* Make sure that you buy pure essential oils from a reputable retailer or pharmacist. Some companies use artificial scents, and these will not have the true benefits of essential oils. It is important to patch test oils first and check for sensitivity 24 hours before using any oil or combination of oils. Oils can also cause skin sensitivity to sunlight. The evidence suggests avoiding aromatherapy when pregnant and breastfeeding. Trust your body. If it doesn't feel right, discontinue.

## Gut love massage

Make your own massage blend – choose the oils, follow your gut. Oils can be stimulants, relaxants or neutral. So select the oils based on the time of day and your stress levels.

1. Create a comfortable place to lie down on a sofa or bed, with a towel or sheet under you if you are worried about oils on clothing or fabric.

2. Complete at least three cycles of base belly breathing (*see page 31*). If you're particularly stressed, toggle your breath with your hands, touch the oil to your nose and inhale deeply into the base of your belly for a few moments before you begin.

3. Take a generous tablespoon of oil and rub it between your hands. Cup your hands to your face first and inhale.

4. Place your hands flat against your stomach with your fingers covering your belly button and start with a soft, wide opening stroke down and outwards. If you can, take your hands around your sides and behind your lower back. Then move upwards slowly across your lower back and kidneys and back to the front of your body. Do this move several times – the key is slowly. Breathe deeply into your belly in a slow rhythm to the movement of your hands.

5. Be as gentle and slow as you can. Then slow down some more. The way you circle the movement of massage around your stomach depends on how often you go to the loo.

    - For IBS (diarrhoea), a super gentle counterclockwise movement may support the slowing down of your digestive tract.

    - For IBS (constipation), you may find a gentle clockwise movement will support you to eliminate.

    - For Crohn's disease, close your eyes and allow your hands to gently massage the higher section of your belly, focusing on your ileum and colon. Focus on those areas where you sense inflammation – be as gentle and loving as possible. Remember, your meds act to mask pain and inflammation, so travel slowly, mindfully over your gorgeous gut.

    - For ulcerative colitis, follow the ascending, transverse, and descending colon with slow, tender movements. Let your hands gently and lovingly sweep around the curve of your colon. Use your two hands to gently complete a large, slow-moving circle.

6. Repeat this gentle pressure for 12 long cycles, go light and then go lighter; only start to add a firm, soft hold if it feels right. Remember you have a lot packed into your abdominal area, and you don't want to cause any additional pressure – your abdomen is three-dimensional. Wrap your hands around your sides, along the lower ribs and upper hips. This will deepen your sense of relaxation and slow your breathing.

7. Deepen your massage by visualizing the shape of your colon, the folds of your ileum. And as you do this, you can visualize healing light, cooling and soothing, moving through them as you massage. You may want to quietly thank them.

8. As you massage, you will naturally feel the expansion of your abdomen area as you breathe. Time the strokes of your hands to support your breath naturally and effortlessly to slow. Remember, if you are in a flare and your belly feels swollen or distended, then simple toggling your hands to the rhythm of your breath on your stomach area can support. Or hold your belly by cupping flat palms lightly over your belly.

9. End by returning your hands to the starting position, thanking yourself for taking the time out of your day to offer your loving attention to your beloved guts.

## *7. Foot care is gut care*

Have you ever noticed your feet in a flare? You may notice the soft fleshy arches of your feet are extra tender. According to reflexology, our whole body exists in our feet, so foot care is essential to self-care and can be a lovely alternative to belly massage.

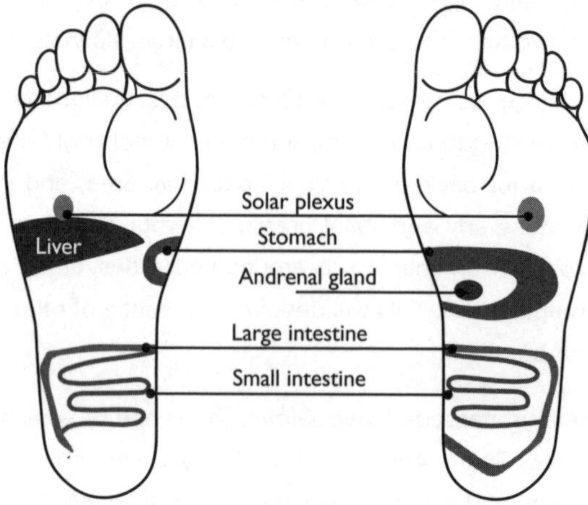


Figure 7: Map of foot health, according to reflexology

Our bodies form a map of our inner world. The body is an interconnected place. If you're having problems with bloating, a good foot massage can do wonders. Just think about it. Our feet get a daily battering. They are tied up for most of the day, too often in pretty uncomfortable shoes. And then trussed up that way they get to carry around all our weight – the whole day long.

## Gut-loving foot massage

This massage is one of the best ways to ensure a restful night's sleep. Combined with base belly breathing, it will see you drift off in no time

1. Get your favourite massage oil and use the thumb and fingers of both hands to clasp the ball of your foot – just below your toes – and press firmly. Your feet carry you around all day; they can take it.

2. Push outwards and much more gently over the top of your foot.

3. Circle around the foot – treat it as fully three-dimensional. Breathe. Move down the foot and repeat, less pressure on the underside of the arch and repeat – it's that simple.

4. Make sure you focus on the arch of the foot. This is where the solar plexus chakra is mapped (*see figure 4, page 30*), and this is also where the large and small intestine is mapped. If you notice tenderness, then reduce pressure and slow down and breathe as you continue to make large and small circular movements.

Remember the vagus nerve? Well, a good foot massage can act to increase vagal tone, as well as help lower blood pressure – the perfect ritual for sleep surrender.

---

To complete Part II, take a few minutes to revisit your gut life letter from Part I; it's now time to write a love letter from your future gorgeous gut to you.

## A love letter from your gut

To ensure this exercise works, you need to give your gut some space and time. Find a quiet place, away from distraction and interruption and take out your Gut-loving Journal.

1. Take deep breaths down into your root chakra (*see figure 4, page 30*). You will find as you continue to take deep base belly breaths that you will naturally energize your solar plexus chakra.

2. Now move your hands to your heart area, and take a few moments to think of someone you love dearly, a person or animal. Choose someone where the emotion is really straightforward and uncomplicated – an aunt, a grandparent, a family pet. Feel that sense of love naturally arise in you. You may feel a sense of light or

warmth rest in that. As you let that feeling fill you, start to connect to the deepest, most loving place within you. If you feel a little stuck, just say aloud, 'I connect to the place of wisdom and compassion that sits right at my centre.'

3. Now pick up your pen and write a letter to yourself from your future self and your gut; choose a time at least five years from now, or be brave and go further into the future, maybe decades from now. Write today's date and add the year you're writing from. So from this future time, you and your gut are writing to your current self. Let your gut thank you for all the changes you have made to honour and heal it.

4. Sign off in the most loving way you can to your current self (acknowledging where you are now) from your future self and healthy gut. Wish them well on the journey, and inspire them with how well your future gut is doing.

---

## GUT COMPASSION

- Time to tone up that vagus nerve (*see page 65*).
- Spend time growing your gut instincts, to shape a more mindful food flow in your weekly shop (*see pages 84 and 86*)
- Practice being present with your plate and creating your very own gut grace (*see page 92*).
- Gut-Shui your room and create new gut-loving rituals for sleep (*see page 96*).

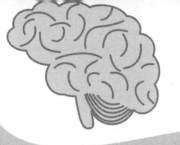

## Part III

# GUT HEALING

***'You have a unique body and mind... Only by listening inwardly in a fresh and open way will you discern at any given time what most serves your healing and freedom.'***

Tara Brach, *True Refuge*

It's time to explore gut-healing foods and how you can make simple changes to reduce the impact of inflammation in your life. We'll explore why it's important to deindustrialize our gorgeous gut and challenge the idea that we're missing out on the foods everyone else is eating, which are no good for us or our dear gut.

You'll shine a light on the inner self-talk and use affirmations to send love to each part of the precious piece of kit that makes up your gut. You'll find compassionate ways to eliminate common trigger foods and gently unravel the fear of flaring in a 10-step flare plan. We'll also explore how to use movement to balance your microbiome, including my favourite technique: the Gut Love Dance.

## Chapter 9

# Eliminate with Love

*'Compassion is the basis of all morality.'*

Arthur Schopenhauer, philosopher

The landscape of the food fads and healthy diets is complex to navigate. Quite a few diets will promise to fix your gut – and maybe they will, but that may not be the whole story. There are so many different kinds of diets, and some will do you and your microbes more harm than good. It can feel a little overwhelming to decide what's right for you and your gut – low histamine, low carb, paleo, soya free, low FODMAP – there are just so many to choose from. The sheer scale of options means you could end up wasting a fair amount of time and effort going down the wrong food path.

Take a breath. We are going to look at some of the best advice out there. But remember you get to choose – that is, you and your gut.

A wise man said a few millennia ago, 'Let food be thy medicine and medicine be thy food.' We've got to hand it to the ancient Greeks; in a pre-scientific world, they knew a thing or two. Our modern take on Hippocrates' words is the oft-quoted phrase 'You are what you eat.' And, of course, what we eat shapes our microbes.

It turns out that the standard Western diet is a villain in our gut health story. A Western industrialized diet tends to have a heavy load of chemical preservatives and high levels of sugar, fat and salt. An elimination diet, therefore, can be the stepping-stone to gut healing – a short-term process usually guided by a nutritionist or dietician. And let's be clear, an elimination diet is not about dieting. Rather it is about creating a **personalized food map** for your gut health.

## Gut Gaia and food choices

There are approximately **30,000 edible plants** on the planet, and we eat around 150 of them.[1] A staggering 50 per cent of global calories come from just three plants: wheat, rice and maize. Philosopher and activist Vandana Shiva asks us to reimagine a world where we talk of 'nutrition or health per acre' rather than the traditional model of 'yield per acre'.[2] Your personal Gut Gaia, and the wider planetary Gaia, are part of a symbiotic dance.

Let's take a deep belly breath and contemplate that for a moment. When you show up to your plate with presence, you've got a clear-sighted line of view. Your individual food choices are a thread in a broad tapestry.

*The global food production system beyond our kitchen cupboards may feel far away, but it's not separate from us.*

So here's a challenge next time you pop to your local supermarket or grocery store. You know the way you always navigate through and pick up the 'usual'. Stop there for a minute and look around you.

### ♥ Gut Love ♥

What new plant-based ingredients could you add to your basket this week? Try this on a Friday or a weekend. Go big or go home! Choose the wackiest ingredient you can find. Feed your darling gut bugs something they've never had their tiny mitts on before.

## The spirit of *Calm Your Gut*

Your human microbiome keeps co-evolving. So time to keep learning about and loving those microbes. Who else will tend to your gut, have compassion for your microbiome, if not you? This is the spirit of *Calm Your Gut*. Our guts are beautifully intelligent, sensitive organs filled with a symphony of bacteria. To make beautiful music, you want the whole orchestra – violins, piano, cello, clarinet, percussion. Yep, you want all of them. And this is the message about diversity – living plant diversity.

On your journey towards gut balance, you may meet folks who swear by a particular diet. Great, if it works for them. But as you've discovered, your IBD and my IBD may look and feel different. We each inhabit the landscape of our own unique flare. Your IBS might be triggered by dairy, mine by wheat. She healed her Crohn's disease with celery juice and apple cider vinegar (ACV). She has crafted a careful FODMAP-based elimination diet to manage her IBS symptoms. He made the difficult decision to have a stoma to heal his body and his gut. That all being said, what is becoming clear is that the evidence is growing that maintaining remission in IBD is supported by a diet rich in pre and probiotic foods.[3]

Our microbiomes are as unique as our individual fingerprints. Therefore, rebalancing and restoring your individual microbiome takes you on a unique healing journey. One in which we can share our highs and lows, our growing wisdom, and celebrate each other along our unique journey.

## Whatever you do, eliminate with LOVE

A successful elimination diet takes a significant commitment and time. It's a changing journey and requires clear-sighted motivation. It will ask compassion and consistency of you in equal measure. When your gut is sore and inflamed, it requires your commitment to gentle, strong healing. Sometimes we can almost overwhelm our bodies by eating such a drastically different diet that it results in confusion and makes our gut off-kilter. So begin where you are – today. Keep it simple. Start small but be consistent in the direction you're taking. What I do know:

*Your loved-up and listened-to gut will offer you some great advice.*

When your actions are shaped by gut knowledge and nourished by your growing gut compassion, you'll find it easier to commit to sustained change. Changing from what most folks are eating around, you will require a daily choice of self-care. In fact, it will ask for fierce and committed compassion from you. This can be tough. One small-scale study by A. Justine Dowd MD[4] on a group of young women with coeliac disease (a condition where the immune system attacks the gut when gluten-based foods are eaten) showed that those with higher self-worth levels managed to follow a gluten-free diet.

This makes sense. Self-compassion is the bridge between what we know and how we act. A deep heartfelt connection to our gut makes it easier to commit and follow through. Some studies on IBS and low FODMAP diet initially floundered because of poor levels of adherence. To buy and prepare unprocessed foods takes effort, one you'll only commit to when you know your gorgeous gut is worth it.

*Self-care is the foundation of sustained change.*

At times you may even have to sit out the occasional food addiction withdrawals. It doesn't necessarily mean you can never eat specific foods ever again, but you may discover some are your personal kryptonite – sugar, dairy, beer. Some foods will trigger your gut no matter what. The good news: find your food kryptonite, and you become empowered to heal your gut. As long as you eat food that triggers an inflammatory response, your guts can't heal. No matter how much celery juice you drink or however many probiotics you take.

## What to reduce

Whatever your health status right now, there is pretty consistent evidence that reducing or removing the following four foods from your life will improve your gut wellbeing and overall health. So take a deep breath into that beautiful belly, and let's see what you need to chuck out of those kitchen cupboards.

### *1. Highly processed foods*

These have undergone processes to add preservatives and chemicals for shelf life. There's growing evidence that highly processed meats are carcinogenic. Most traditional junk food is highly processed. If you're a junk-food addict, it's time to take action to reduce, reframe and rediscover some alternatives this week.

## *2. Sugar*

It's time to wean yourself off the white (and brown) stuff because sugar is in the inflammatory food group. There are fair few politics in the sugar lobby, so if you are a sugar addict, I really encourage you to learn more. Knowing more about sugar will drive your motivation and transform what you see as a 'treat' into something you know is addictive and no good for your beloved gut. The average British person eats around 28kg (62lb) of sugar a year.[5] For the average American, it's more than double that at 69kg (152lb) a year. Wow, that's a whole lot of sugar.

Sugar can hide in the most unexpected places, with labels like corn syrup, maltose and glucose etc. So how can you **reduce** the burden of the sweet stuff? Well, a little creativity goes a long way. I have a hard and fast rule that I either **replace** or **reduce** in recipes. However, you'll need to step away from artificial sweeteners, too (so look out for aspartame, sucralose or saccharin). There's growing evidence of the potential health hazards of artificial sweeteners, including increased inflammation and damage to our microbiome. So time to replace and rediscover natural forms of sugar, such as maple syrup, date sugar and stevia, which are good natural substitutes or quality, local sourced honey in moderation can help wean you off the sweet stuff.

## *3. Refined carbohydrates*

These are common forms of processed foods and deserve a special mention as they are usually quick, easy, addictive stuff: white bread, pasta, pastries and pizza. You may need to *reframe* your thinking around these foods. They are often laced with an addictive sugar and/or salt combo. So time to **reduce, replace and rediscover** healthy, homemade alternatives. (In Part V, I share some quick and easy alternatives in my beat-the-bloat recipes, including traditional gluten-free, dairy-free and yeast-free soda bread, which is my go-to).

### *4. Emulsifiers*

These tend to hide in plain sight and include **trans** and **partially hydrogenated fats**. Also, polyunsaturated fats in margarine, processed foods and oils. If you don't recognize the words on your food packaging, and it sounds chemical, they are likely to be food preservatives. Whole, freshly cooked foods don't contain them. Most pre-packed, pre-prepared foods with a long shelf life do. Recent research on the microbiome reveals that some common emulsifiers may actually thin the mucosal lining of your gut.[6] Try cooking without oil – surprisingly easy for most meals. If you have to, if you need to, then try adding a little water to reduce the temperature of the heated oil. A little bit of coconut oil used sparingly is among the better choices, as it is resistant to oxidation at high heat compared to most other oils.

*Your new mantra: Reduce, replace, reframe, rediscover.*

As you reprogramme your gut and your mindset, you'll surely have times when you feel like you're missing out. And well, yes, that may be the case. So as you turn towards new food choices, focus on the positive choices you *can* eat – time for a little creativity and experimentation.

## CHAPTER 10

# THE RESILIENT GUT

*'If you think you're too busy to take care of yourself, you're eventually going to be too sick to be busy.'*

BROOKE GOLDNER, PHYSICIAN AND AUTHOR

If you're on a quest to eliminate certain foods, you might be wondering about the best diets for good gut health. An elimination diet may not resolve every gut symptom, but it will certainly play a part in your healing. It's like setting your internal reset button. Giving your body a vacation from specific foods enables it to stop the inflammation cycle, enabling your gut's mucosal lining to repair. Your gut will become less sensitive, less swollen and less inflamed.

A good elimination diet is a bit like the lead-up to a successful political campaign. You'll need to plan in advance, get your publicity right, write your gut manifesto and stick to it. Stressful work situations or an ill child can derail your efforts. Christmas, Passover, Thanksgiving, your spouse's birthday – all of these occasions can undo plans. So the trick is to plan and then plan some more. Once you start, you need to have a fierce, loving, compassionate commitment to keep following through.

*Self-compassion is the bridge between our knowledge and action.*

## Elimination diets

Remember, we and our microbes are addicts. When we stop eating the usual high-sugar, refined carbs, we'll starve those particular gut bugs. To make it easier, you might choose to follow a tried-and-tested elimination diet. Let's take a look at a few.

## Low FODMAP

The undisputed queen of IBS diets is the low FODMAP diet. So just what is it? FODMAP stands for fermentable oligosaccharides, disaccharides, monosaccharides and polyols. The main dietary sources of the four groups of FODMAPs to avoid include:[7]

- Oligosaccharides: Wheat, rye, specific fruits and some specific vegetables, including the allium family: garlic and onions.
- Disaccharides: Milk, including dairy-based cheese and yoghurt.
- Monosaccharides: Specific fruits like figs, mango and sweeteners such as honey and agave nectar.
- Polyols: Specific fruits and vegetables like mushrooms and stone fruits. They are also found in products like sugar-free gum and some diabetic sweeteners.

The low FODMAP diet has shown success in around 80–85 per cent of IBS sufferers who've tried it. The essential diet is based on an eight-week programme with a clear dietary plan. It's specialist and specific, and you may need to get support from a registered dietician and follow trusted recipe guidance. Adherence rates are low, as it is a little complicated to get your head around. To ensure success, you will need to have built a good foundation in gut knowledge and gut compassion.

The low FODMAP diet is ***not*** a lifestyle diet to be sustained for a long time. Rather it is a short period of excluding certain food triggers. Many of the excluded foods are crucial to good gut health, including the allium family (garlic) and apples (ACV). The plan is a careful reintroduction of the foods to support you to have a diverse diet. The irrepressibly energetic brothers Dave and Steve, creators of 'The Happy Pear', have created some great plant-based courses. See the Resources section for useful links.

## Food combining and an Ayurvedic approach

There is a lot of sense in the concept of food combining, and you may even have some instincts for a particular set of foods, which when eaten together cause you to feel bloated and uncomfortable. Take a note of this, be curious and attuned to your gut talk.

Avoid too much fluid intake during eating. If you have a digestive health concern, you may already have low levels of key enzymes. By gulping down water during a meal, you will further dilute these key parts of food's chemical breakdown.

I have a particular affinity with the Ayurvedic approach. It is based on an ancient wisdom tradition, which focuses on supporting balance in the body rather than distinct symptomatology. Deepak Chopra's *Perfect Healing*[8] is a great starting point for further exploration. In Ayurvedic medicine, the aim is to create balance in the three *doshas* – *vatta*, *pitta* and *kapha* – (air, fire and earth) to understand your body type. Those of us with digestive health issues often have an imbalance in our *pitta* (fire) *dosha* – too much or too little. The premise is to seek balance, to restore homeostasis in the body, mind and spirit through diet and lifestyle.

One of Ayurvedic medicine's key premises is to ensure your main meal is around the midpoint of the day when your digestive fire (*pitta*) is at its peak, but also to tweak your eating patterns to support balance in your *doshas*. The approach is about tuning into the wider circadian (24-hour) rhythms of your body and enabling you to adjust to seasonal changes, which significantly impact the body and digestion.

The pre-scientific world's underlying intuition based on creating balance in the body is ancient gut wisdom at its best. In our more sophisticated world where we diagnose and treat health differently, the body–mind is rarely seen as an integrated whole. If you are curious about non-Western approaches to diet, go with your gut and find the right practitioner for you.

Check out Ananta Ripa Ajmera at www.theancientway.co for further inspiration on an Ayurvedic approach to eating.

## Plant-based

There is a growing movement towards plant-based, vegan diets. A plant-based diet certainly aligns with wider respect for the global Gaia. Plant-based is my preference. I make rare instinct-led deviations from plant-based foods.

A word of caution: to eat a healthy, balanced plant-based diet takes a little skill and commitment to ensure sufficient access to complete proteins, micronutrients like vitamin B-complex and iron. If you are currently dealing with a flare, always seek advice from your medical team and dietitian/nutritionist. But also trust the growing wisdom of your gut. Our ancestors used gut wisdom to combine incomplete proteins to create a complete protein source like rice and black beans, hummus and oatcakes, quinoa and cruciferous veg. These types of combinations can also make the plant form of protein more bioavailable. An example of this is turmeric – the active anti-inflammatory compound curcumin is more available for absorption when cooked with black pepper – just as it is used in traditional Indian cuisine.

My early days as an unhealthy teen vegetarian almost certainly negatively impacted my microbiome. My diet then was limited, so my gut bugs were excited to see the move towards diverse, healthy plant-based diets which skilfully combine varied plant sources. Gut knowledge and collective gut wisdom are growing globally. We now know the best approach is to combine prebiotics and probiotics: this would look like quinoa (high protein, high fibre) with sauerkraut (probiotic), or brown rice (high fibre) with a side order of fermented kimchi (probiotic). I share some of my go-to recipes in Part V.

## The Mediterranean diet

The Mediterranean diet has shown wide-ranging health benefits consistently. Sometimes called the anti-inflammatory diet, it focuses on a diet rich in varied plants, fish, nuts, legumes and some meat. The aim is to eat a diverse range of plant-based foods and focus on olive oil, the allium family (garlic, onion) and prebiotics (e.g. artichokes). It is a diet marked by balance, variety and regular consumption of a small amount of polyphenol-rich red wine each day.

It's now very clear that we all have a responsibility to reduce our animal products intake[9] because meat production is bad for the environment. The Mediterranean diet offers a balance focusing on plants with a small proportion of fish and meat.

There are a few specialist IBD diets, and these may support people with diverticulitis and coeliac disease, as well as easing symptoms and supporting remission in ulcerative colitis and Crohn's disease.

## Specific Carbohydrate Diet (SCD)

The SCD was originally created in the early 20th century by Dr Sydney Hass and developed further by biochemist Elaine Gottschall in the 1980s in response to her daughter's severe ulcerative colitis. This diet focuses on removing grains, starches, processed and canned food. There is a focus on fresh fruit and veg, meat and dairy are included, and homemade yoghurt is used to feed your good gut bugs. The anecdotal evidence is that many folks with IBD and also children with autism have benefitted from this diet. There are no large-scale controlled studies to support some evidence for improved symptoms – and the diet can be hard to stick to. However with the ever-increasing availability of a wide-selection of dietary alternatives, plus some great online support groups, this diet can be a viable option.

## IBD Anti-inflammatory Diet (IBD-AID)

The IBD-AID has evolved from the SCD, incorporating the latest research on the microbiome to include pre- and probiotics as a core element of the gut-healing process. The diet recognizes that the balance of gut bugs in those with IBD is different – that's the starting point. The aim is to reduce inflammation and support the microbiome's balance through a gradual phasing of foods. The Director of the Center for Applied Nutrition at UMass Medical School, Barbara Olendzki, created the IBD-AID. The research and small-scale studies continue to support the understanding of this diet's impact even with those who have severe flares. This diet deserves a special mention because there is a wealth of science behind it.

Therefore, the diet follows guidance on removing inflammatory foods and monitoring symptoms. To give you a brief overview: the IBD-AID diet is based around a three-phase approach to introducing foods, and emphasizes avoiding certain carbohydrates that are pro-inflammatory, which may be disturbing the normal gut flora. Foods that contain lactose, wheat, refined sugar (sucrose) and corn are avoided in all phases of the diet. The theory goes:

- Avoidance can starve out the bad bacteria.
- Avoidance of these foods helps a sensitive gut recover.
- Eliminating trans fats (store-bought baked goods, anything containing partially hydrogenated oil), processed foods and fast food can help to restore the lining of the gut wall.[10]

OK, I've saved the best till last, so I hope you're paying attention. The IBD-AID is the one that my personal food map most closely aligns with my own evolving gut-led diet. Alongside avoiding wheat, I also avoid corn – a common ingredient in many free-from products. But I encourage you to follow your gut-led wisdom every time in your own approach.

## Fad diets, healing diets and medical mainstream thinking

Traditionally mainstream medical thinking worries about elimination diets. An understandable concern is that those of us living with chronic health conditions could be making ad hoc decisions to remove key food groups from our diet. In fact, when we flare, we have an increased risk of malnutrition and a low BMI.

I speak from experience. As I described earlier in the book, at the lowest point of my health journey, my BMI was a dangerous 16. The NHS dietician and gastro consultant looked unhappy when I shared my intention to stop eating gluten. This was the early 2000s. At that time, the mainstream wisdom for IBD was a traditional low-fibre, low-residue diet. We now know that whilst this may form part of the traditional treatment protocol for a flare, it is not the best approach to treating IBD. In fact, a low-fibre diet may even 'accelerate dysbiosis in IBD'.[11]

There has to be sensible caution about approaching an elimination diet. You need to be at a point in your healing journey where you have a degree of stability to embark on a meaningful elimination diet. When there are too many varying factors, for example, changes in your meds or your lifestyle, it can be extremely hard to (1) sustain an elimination diet and (2) unravel the impact of that diet. That being said, if you are unwell, avoid known trigger foods. Aim to reduce your intake of the top four inflammatory triggers: sugar, highly processed foods, emulsifiers and refined carbs (*see page 119*).

**Gluten and dairy** are two of the most widespread foods to which many of us instinctively feel we have an intolerance. They are on-trend, and for many of us with IBD and IBS, we may get some immediate symptom relief by removing them, but it may not be the whole story. Gluten-free is not a byword for healthy so beware of some of the free-from products out there. There are some wonderful, creative brands, a few of which I've listed in the Resources (*see page 266*).

However, there are also some pretty unhealthy things on the shelves of some of the major supermarkets. The big brands and the supermarkets have been playing catch-up with the huge (and no doubt lucrative) demand of free-from that's come from more and more of us stepping away from the mainstream, as we begin to understand the impact of certain foods on our guts, bodies and minds. But if the response of the brands and shops is often motivated by profit margins (as appears likely), it's not always helping out our guts.

It's been a time of experimentation, and much of the free-from thinking is 'how do we create a free-from product with shelf life and taste?' Sound familiar? It was that kind of mindset that led to the Chorleywood baking method. When wheat disappears, there's a lot of corn (which is a common GMO food). Some products are second-rate versions of the mainstream food items with extra sugar, extra emulsifiers, etc. The shelf life and lip life of food don't equate to good gut health. The two are frequently opposed.

So slow down and step warily around the packaging. Don't assume free-from equates to healthy. Unfortunately, it's not that simple. What we are seeking to do is to protect the health of our beautifully diverse (strong yet fragile) microbiomes. This work is crucial for our guts and our waistlines.

## Gut-healing foods

So how do you navigate the long list of diets to commit to your own personalized food map? Well, the science is pointing us towards some interesting areas. It's an ever-evolving picture.

*Hold the science in one hand and get a firm hold of your gut in the other.*

### *Gut healing in six steps*

1. **Eat for colour:** We know in the UK that it's five a day. In fact, the research suggests it's more likely eight-plus. There's undisputed evidence of the health benefits of eating a plant-based diet and of upping your daily and weekly intake of veg and fruit for wellbeing. The different colours equate to different phytonutrients, so seek out your own food rainbow. If you currently don't eat many vegetables, start slowly and increase gradually. A simple way to increase your intake is to mix up a morning fruit-and-veg smoothie. Easy on the gut and a great way of starting your day off with three or four plant-based ingredients.

2. **Fibre-fuelled diversity:** Aim for at least 30 different sources of fibre. Fibre is a total sweetheart for your microbiome, and we are not eating nearly enough – an average of 10–15g against an ideal of 30g or more. If you are healing or in a flare, go slowly and keep a diary or **food mood tracker** (*see page 133*) – aim to increase your fibre intake over weeks or even months.

3. **Eat organic when you can:** Eating organic is costly, so if you are on a budget, be discerning. Small grains like brown rice, quinoa and oats have a large cumulative surface area – meaning pesticides

can accumulate in them, so aim for organic when you can. Where you can't, be mindful of how you wash and prepare foods. A cheap way to up your access to organic produce is to grow your own fruit, herbs and veg. Growing your own has another added bonus. In an allotment or garden, you can get your hands in the soil and get to breathe in your biome (#breatheyourmicrobiome).

4. **Keep it simple:** Rediscover the unprocessed, whole foods your grandparents ate. If you glance at the listed ingredients and need a PhD in chemistry to understand what you're eating, then put it back.

5. **Eat good fats:** Olive oil (ideally cold-pressed, extra virgin), avocados (if not low FODMAP), whole organic butter. These foods can nourish your gut's delicate lining and contain butyric acid – your gut-loving healing friend.

6. **Fast:** Make sure you give your gut a break by fasting overnight and occasionally for 14–16 hours. Fasting is pretty simple. Don't eat late in the evening and aim to eat breakfast later so your gut is not working a long shift. Your gut needs a break too. When we graze all day, we can create something called postprandial inflammation – the natural rise in digestive inflammation after eating.

OK, so far, so good – all doable, yep? Healing is always going to be an inside job. The body has incredible healing powers, but it also has rules of engagement, rules of care. As Lao Tzu said: 'A journey of a thousand miles begins with a single step.'

To support your success, I recommend creating a **food mood tracker**. This will help you become the detective of your own gorgeous gut health by unravelling how different foods impact your gut. If you are taking a high dose of meds, this can mask some of your reactions, so you will need to look out for subtle signs. This includes the obvious – bloating, gas, a subtle sense of inflammation or increased loo visits. Look out for wider symptoms: a sense of irritation, brain fog or low energy.

You can buy a journal or create your own in a notebook. Take a ruler and draw four lines down the page. I've given you some ideas below about useful headings. I've purposely tried to keep the what and the how separate, as you'll be surprised how often what can have a different outcome depending on how you show up to your plate.

Once you've got your food mood tracker ready to go, it's useful to record in it over a short period at first to get used to the process. You may even spot trends in how your body and gut are rapidly responding to certain foods – or it may be a little slower and more complex to unravel. Just remember, some of your very best gut-loving knowledge can come from this practice.

| Food Mood Tracker | | | |
|---|---|---|---|
| What you ate | How you ate: | How you felt immediately after eating: | How you felt 24–48 hours after eating: |
| Err... the full honest account. Who are you kidding? | On the run, mindfully, and any place in between. | This is where the 'what' and 'how' will help you make sense of any symptoms of bloating or discomfort. | How you generally feel, sleep, mood, physical reactions.<br>Of course, at this stage also how it goes through you.<br>You might want to note here any specific external factors – a job interview, deadline etc. |

This little food diary is going to be a gold mine of information for you and also for your gut gang – your IBD nurse consultant. A tool to decode your unique gut responses. I'd also suggest jotting down any reflections and helpful tips for yourself. Keep it simple but keep it updated, even if you miss a meal or a day. This notebook is a place for you to self-coach and self-care. Get curious about your plate. If you know (and sometimes you just do) something triggers you, honour your gut and avoid it. Remember, it might not be forever, but avoid it while you're still unravelling your food kryptonite. So leave it alone, however much you feel you can't live without it.

If you're struggling to unravel your triggers, you may also want to get a blood test for IgG. However, the scientific accuracy of these tests remains unclear. If you have intestinal permeability this may help you to unravel the complex combination of food triggers, but the best plan is an elimination diet supported by a qualified nutritionist or dietician.

## Dysbiosis and flare plan

When we are healthy, our microbiome is resilient – it's a dynamic environment. Alongside diet, many things can trigger an imbalance: excessive alcohol, pollutants, poor sleep, stress and antibiotics, so let's look at some of those in a little more detail.

### *Alcohol – just a little bit*

Studies have been pretty consistent in saying that a small amount of red wine regularly provides increased polyphenols. (I'm known to quote this stat at my local pub.) It is, of course, about balance and, if you are flaring and you've not yet resolved your leaky gut, it is probably best to avoid alcohol altogether. Excessive alcohol can be a cause of intestinal permeability, and it can also disrupt our gut flora balance. So if in doubt, leave it out.

## ♥ Gut Love ♥

Like a glass of red with a meal? Red wine contains health benefiting polyphenols. A glass with dinner lowers the inflammatory marker C-reactive protein. But take it easy, drink in moderation and monitor how it sits with you and your gut.

### *Create an anti-inflammatory lifestyle*

OK, let's just take a moment to widen the lens of gut healing. The evidence suggests we need to create a more anti-inflammatory lifestyle. This includes getting sufficient sleep, reducing stress, and including movement and exercise. In the journey towards the calm gut, we explore all of these. To further reduce inflammation, we can:

#### Reduce exposure to chemicals

It turns out city living is a risk for our gut microbes. We're surrounded by a cocktail of chemical pollutants: traffic, pesticides, cleaning products. A fair few studies suggest air pollution is a factor in the development of IBD.[12] What we can exert a measure of control over is the sphere of our homes. Consider ditching the non-stick pans for old fashioned steel pans or green frying pans. If you can invest in a pressure cooker – a great way of cooking pulses like chickpeas and legumes at speed – you can reduce your use of tinned food and the burden of bisphenol A (BPA) in your diet. Bisphenol A has been shown to disrupt the body's endocrine system and have a wide range of potential impacts on wellbeing. Cooking with filtered water will help reduce your exposure to some heavy metal residues – aim to change your filter regularly.

When seeking to reduce your exposure to chemicals in your home, start with products in your kitchen and bathroom. If you feel a little overwhelmed, prioritize those products that directly contact your body and food preparation surfaces – deodorants, creams and washing-up products.

### Look after your oral microbiome

Practise good oral hygiene. Your gums are an access point for bacteria into your system. Seek out a healthy toothpaste that is biome-friendly and have regular dental check-ups.

### Green space

If you live in a busy built-up area, plan regular time in green spaces. This is proven to improve physical and mental health. Ecologist and indigenous woman of wisdom Robin Wall Kimmerer's studies reveal 'the smell of humus soil exerts a physiological effect on humans... [and] stimulates the release of (feel-good hormone) oxytocin.'[13] Why not try out a little forest bathing by resting among trees and nature – a few moments create deep calm.

## *Antibiotic action plan*

We know that life-saving courses of antibiotics can be pretty indiscriminate; they kill off the gorgeous lovelies in our guts as well as the bad bugs. There are a few things you can do during and after taking a course to get your glorious guts back on track. As always, prevention is better than cure. A depleted microbiome may leave you more vulnerable to a flare, so try to avoid antibiotics. Be guided by your doctor, but always ask if it's the only way to tackle an infection. As you'll know, we live in a world of increased antibiotic-resistant bacteria, so most GPs are pretty cautious about signing out prescriptions. If you have to take a course, take the best kind of care of yourself and your gut, and you'll soon get back to the best version of yourself.

Consider supplementing a balanced diet with probiotics such as kefir but try and schedule this at different times from the antibiotic tablets.[14] Once the course is over, keep actively eating prebiotics and, of course, supplement with probiotics. Remember, most probiotics tend to be limited to a small number of key strains, and our individual microbiome is uniquely diverse. Post-course, invest time in self-care, get outside and breathe in your biome, and eat the best foods to restore your good gut microbes.

Remember, however sophisticated the current probiotic supplement or pill may be, it's generally the eco-diversity equivalent to a field of oilseed rape in the complex rainforest of our gut. The good news is that there is definite evidence that probiotics have some benefit in IBD outcomes.[15] The pop-a-pill probiotics industry is a billion-dollar business. But there are so many ways to increase your gut lovelies through diet. Over this decade, we will almost certainly have bespoke creations of probiotic bacteria strains, which are unique to our genes and our gut health, although we're not quite there yet.

## The resilient gut

A healthy microbiome is resilient – our bacteria levels wax and wane for a host of reasons. The aim is to build up your underlying level of resilience by supporting the diversity of your microbes. As you know, many of us with IBD and IBS are likely experiencing a form of imbalance in our gut, our very own personal dysbiosis.

The idea that healing is a single event has an appeal, but in my experience, it is an ongoing journey. With your unique dysbiosis, you may find it takes a little time to restore your wellbeing. At first, the balance may be a little fragile and easily disrupted, but slowly,

slowly, as you build resilience, the varied species grow, and you create an ecosystem that becomes a self-sustaining home.

Re-establishing your microbiome is a dance, a journey. It is strong and fragile, just like us. If we gift it each day with the right fuel, we can bring it home little by little. When I undertook my microbiome mapping, I chatted to the inspiring Hay House author, Shann Nix Jones (aka CEO of Chuckling Goat). She shared a story that really stuck with me from the indigenous wisdom of the Cherokee people:

> *A grandfather told his grandson, you have two wolves inside of you. One is harsh, greedy and full of hate. The other is kind, generous and caring. The grandson asked. 'But grandfather, how do I get rid of the bad wolf?' and the grandfather said: 'You feed the good wolf'.*

So, what does it mean to feed the good wolf?

## Feeding those gorgeous gut bugs the 3Ps

It's time to get to know your probiotics, prebiotics and polyphenols. Then you can start to build these into your day and week. In simple terms, **probiotics** mean increasing the number of friendly bugs in your gut. **Prebiotics** help feeds those gut bugs, so they thrive. **Polyphenols** are packed with varied micronutrients that help you to function.

### *Probiotics*

As we understand more and more about gut bugs, we can start to focus on the bacteria, which reduce inflammation and repair the lining of the gut wall. These include lactobacillus and bifidobacterium bacteria, like the lovely lactobacillus acidophilus. So try eating:

- Kefir – goat's kefir for vegetarians and coconut-based kefir for vegans

- Sauerkraut – pickled cabbage, easy to make and full of good gut bugs
- Kimchi – fermented cabbagy goodness for your gut
- Live yoghurt – (watch out for added sugar)
- Probiotic pills – good-quality probiotics have shown clinical improvements in IBD and especially ulcerative colitis. Take a supplement for a period but nourish these gut bugs, food first.

### *Prebiotics*

There's a real buzz around fermented foods right now because our lovely gut bugs can feast on fermented goodies. Homemade is simple and effective, and you can adapt the recipe to your palate. I love caraway seeds in my homemade fermented goodies. Remember, diverse plant-based fibre is a great prebiotic for replenishing friendly lovelies like bifidobacteria and lactobacilli.[16]

- Artichoke[17] or Jerusalem artichoke
- Asparagus
- Green bananas
- Alliums, like garlic, leeks, onions
- Chicory – high in gut-loving inulin

### *Polyphenols*

Polyphenols contain micronutrients that support digestive health, so pack your diet with a range of polyphenols each day. Some of the best are:

- Green tea – full of bonus phytonutrients and lower in caffeine (black tea is good too)

- Berries, in particular, blueberries
- Herbs like cloves and peppermint
- Nuts like pecans and hazelnuts
- Dark chocolate (85 per cent plus)
- Cacao nibs – great in flapjacks or for an indulgent hot chocolate
- Grapes are a great source; red wine in moderation may be beneficial

So how can you plan your week with the 3Ps in mind? Every time you decide to act in a way that aligns with your gut health needs, you are taking a step towards true gut integrity. You are aligning with your internal Gut Gaia. As you honour your gut and commit to its care, you'll find that your gut instinct grows stronger; it signifies you are moving towards an authentic gut-led life.

**♥ Gut Love ♥**

Keep on growing that gut-loving wisdom. As your intuition grows, it will speak to you more and more.

## Pharmanutrition for gut health

OK, you've started to put the foundations in place by removing four of the most common inflammatory foods and including more of the 3Ps. There's a whole world of fibre and fermented foods just waiting to nurture your gut. Some of the good stuff is listed below. This list isn't exhaustive – just a few ways to gut-loving care.

### *Gut fibre loving*

- Chia seeds – queen of fibre and protein
- Psyllium husk[18] – simple to stir into some porridge (my fave!)
- Flaxseed – especially good for anyone needing to boost phytoestrogens
- Dandelion leaves[19] – the delicate early leaves are best to add to salads
- Legumes – chickpeas, black beans, adzuki, boleti
- Lentils – easy for curries and flatbreads
- Whole grains – quinoa, brown rice, millet, buckwheat
- Oats – a great source of soluble fibre, even better, steel-cut oats
- Cruciferous crunch – broccoli, sprouts, cauliflower, cabbage, kale

### *Fermented foods*

- Apple cider vinegar (ACV) – unpasteurized and organic, great in salad dressing
- Seaweed – miso paste stirred into wholesome soups
- Sauerkraut – add a tangy dollop on the side of your plate
- Kombucha – easy to make at home as a tea or soft drink
- Tempeh – fermented soy

### *Omega-rich foods*

- Olive oil – go for cold-pressed quality and drizzle over bread and pasta

- Avocado – breakfast/brunch favourite, and it can add a creamy texture to desserts
- Nuts and nut butter – an extra protein on the side of your plate
- Flaxseeds – easy additions to smoothies, yoghurt, bread and breakfasts

## How does this compare to your current food map?

I hope you're feeling inspired – but maybe you're searching this list for some of your favourite foods. Ahem, so let's just take stock for a minute. Our standard Western diet is designed to create cravings, trigger dopamine and get us hooked. Ask: who is benefiting? Because let's just be really honest, we're not. And as much as not eating that stuff may *feel* like deprivation, the truth is, it's a gift to you and your gut. This is about a big reframe. We have agency. We have a choice. We get to decide. OK, there's some fierce compassion right there.

Let's pan out again. To commit to your very own deindustrialized gut, let's put the modern diet into context. In the blink of an eye in our microbiome's evolution, 12,000 years ago, humans started cultivating crops after a millennium of hunter-gather diversity.[20] This heralded a big change for our guts.

Fast forward, and in the mid-twentieth century, 60 per cent of the UK's working-age men had a hot homecooked lunch as their main meal. In Ayurvedic nutrition, lunch is the pivot point, when *pitta*, our digestive fire, is at its zenith (*see page 125*) – a place to fill up on warming wholesome food to take us through the rest of our day.

Fast forward again, and in the last 60 years, we find that our ancient digestive tract is facing rapid and radical change. Our diet is vastly different from our pre-crop ancestors and becoming increasingly homogenised around a limited range of grains. I recommend reading Dr David Perlmutter's *Grain Brain*, as he gives a fascinating overview of the impact of this on our gut. Nearly one in five women in the UK suffer from IBS,[21] and we know IBD is also spreading. For those of us with a predisposition to IBD or IBS, we may inadvertently create the perfect conditions for dysbiosis, which can be life-altering or life-limiting. So we need to ask – why? What's going on?

So let's just flip the whole thing about. Is Big Food actually feeding the unfriendly bugs in our gut? Are we undergoing a kind of collective evolutionary Western gut dysbiosis?[22] Is it now time to plan our food with our microbiome in mind?

In countries with strong food cultures, you notice the older shoppers feel the firmness of an avocado or smell the ripeness of local cheese, displaying deep instincts for food. Instincts go flabby with disuse. Preparing food is a gut-life skill. Eating and preparing what we eat with love is a profound act of self-compassion.

## Eliminate with love

An elimination diet is a part of creating an anti-inflammatory environment in your life. These are the steps:

1. **Remove** the inflammatory triggers – diet and chemical pollutants.
2. Slowly and consistently reduce inflammatory foods: sugar and refined carbs.
3. **Reframe** your thinking – this is a biggie for sustainable change. This is not about depriving yourself. This is pure gut-loving care.
4. Aim to repair your gut wall – that beautiful mucosal barrier is protecting your gut. So increase foods that support the synthesis of butyric acid.

5. **Replace** your old inflammatory triggers with a rich, diverse range of plant-based fibre.

6. **Rediscover your gut wisdom** – let it guide your food choices. Plan meals around the 3Ps to repopulate your biome.

*Whatever you do, eliminate with love.*

# CHAPTER 11

# HEALING THE FEAR IN FLARE

*'Everything in your life is there as a vehicle for your transformation. Use it.'*

RAM DASS, SPIRITUAL TEACHER AND AUTHOR

What happens when things aren't going well? Everyone with IBD and IBS knows about flare and fear. We've all been there. So you're in a flare. Your instinct is fear (flares can take many shapes and sizes, from mild bloating to full-on inflammation and pain. If you are living with IBD, then you'll need to be super proactive).

How can we transform the fear of flare? Let's take stock with some practical steps:

1. Alert your gut gang (we'll talk more in the next chapter about creating a resilient gut gang to support you). For now, send a ripple in the wave: email, phone and connect with those who know you and your gut the best. Don't pretend it's not happening, if it is. That's not positive thinking but self-

delusion. But whilst being clear-eyed and absolutely clear-minded – be positive.

2. More specifically, contact your first point medical line: your IBD nurse, GP or consultant, and let them know your symptoms (depending on your history and severity of symptoms). Be proactive.

3. Then, if you're working with an alternative practitioner, nutritionist or dietitian, get in contact and let them know what's happening.

4. Always tell the people who love you – keep your gut health network in the loop. When you're well, give them these questions to ask when you're in flare:

    - What can we do to help?
    - How can I support you today, this week, over the next month with your symptoms?

Get them to keep asking you. The power of those simple questions can carry you far. And if you don't have a good listener in your life, I would encourage you to seek one out. Also, don't overlook the power of learning to ask yourself and your gut those questions calmly and lovingly. There is something powerful about learning to listen deeply to your gut. Your gut holds the wisdom of ages. Give it space, and it will pay you back with gut-loving truths that will shape your life.

OK, so now you've set all that in motion. What can you do for yourself if your gut is in trouble?

## 10 steps to heal your flare

1. Breathe deeply. There are so many benefits to breathing deeply into your belly. You know it supports your vagus because it signals your body to go into rest-and-repair mode. You need this right now. Deep breathing also acts as an inner massage for your gut. There are so many techniques, from the wonderful Wim Hof to Breathworks – explore. Experiment. #breatheyourbiome.

2. Right now, do your gut a favour and slow down. Help your gut out by chewing thoroughly. Be really present with your plate. Choose foods wisely – the foods you are gut-drawn to. Keep asking yourself as you eat: 'What is the work I am asking of my gut right now?' Don't see this as a weight-loss opportunity. That's the wrong mindset and if a loved one has that mindset, challenge yourself and them with fierce, compassionate gut love. That's a dangerous approach to both IBD and IBS. You want to be strong and healthy.

3. Keep a symptom log and food diary. Avoid inflammatory foods. No exceptions – this is no time for the 'just screw it' mentality. Sometimes when we are low in energy, we crave sugar and fat; we are hardwired to. But we know better. These are just the foods to further inflame our gut and create bloating and discomfort.

4. Hydrate with plenty of water and a soothing gut smoothie each morning. These can be simple, tasty ways of keeping up your calories and the range of micronutrients you need. They are best on an empty stomach at the start of the day. Mix in a sprinkle of healing collagen powder (for gut wall repair)

or natural anti-inflammatory powders – boswellia serrata or slippery elm – to pack an extra healing punch. Go easy on the seeds and nuts if this is a trigger.

5. Aim to have a beautiful broth for lunch. Go with your gut and your ethical beliefs. Chicken soup with bones is nourishing with gut-healing collagen. Vegetarian and vegan versions can be supplemented with collagen powder and probiotic miso for tasty extra-fermented goodness. Add anti-inflammatory herbs like turmeric during the cooking process.

6. Amid a flare, avoid alcohol. Yes, I know that may be tough, but your inflamed and bloated guts will thank you for it. Seek out soft healing foods; well-cooked, steamed, gentle, kind foods that you know will help support your internal healing. There are many healing food protocols on offer, including low FODMAP for IBS and IBD-AID. The IBD-AID phase 1 diet is specifically designed for anyone with ulcerative colitis or Crohn's disease who's experiencing an active flare, to ensure that foods are easily absorbed and metabolize without causing irritation. Go with your gut – but be ready to tweak to meet your specific gut needs. Over time and practice, I have found some surprising foods trigger me. So my personal food map is unique and tailored to me.

7. Get plenty of rest and look at ways to ensure healthy sleep at night. Our bodies are hard-wired to the diurnal rhythms of light and dark, and you want to honour your gut bugs. Get as much natural morning light as you can. Do gentle stretches and yoga. Yes, even if you feel awful, the gentlest stretches will help you to reconnect with your tired body and heal. Mindful movements such as yoga, qi gong and tai chi are at heart spiritual exercises, which can bring your heart, head and gut into alignment.

8. Eat food first, but supplement sensibly with support. It is common for those of us with IBD to have difficulty absorbing our B vitamins. So if you're in a flare, an easily absorbable liquid form of B complex under your tongue can be ideal for boosting energy. You may also need to be aware of your iron levels.

9. Eat Japanese style *hara hachi bu*, which means until you are around 80 per cent full. This helps your digestive tract process your food and ensures you are not overfull and bloated.

10. Above all, be kind to yourself. Create yourself a flare gut-love box. In this box, keep your comfy jogging bottoms. You know, the cosy kind that fit over a bloated belly. This can also be where you keep your gut love letter, gut-loving affirmations written in the most beautiful font, a pack of colourful sticky notes that you can place around the house where you can write little reminders to 'breathe' or 'eat slowly' and your favourite belly-rub massage oil. Keep here whatever you need to inspire your healing.

There's one final thing you might wish to consider, and that is taking cannabidiol (CBD) or low dose naltrexone (LDN).[23] There is some emerging evidence about the impact of CBD oil and specifically palmitoylethanolamide (PEA) on supporting the healing of leaky gut.[24] Whilst wide-scale controlled studies have yet to be completed, the anecdotal evidence appears to support the control of pain and many symptoms in IBD and IBS.

Now you're working with your medical team, and you've created some calm. Keep listening. In our modern-day world, where everyone is fighting for some air space and screen time, deep listening is a revolutionary act.

*Listening is critical to your healing.*

Now let's turn within to do the real work. Don't rush through this. If you have never learned to listen to yourself, your body and your gut, and want to heal, now is the time to learn.

## Listening to yourself

There are two beautifully simple ways to start this: journalling and mindfulness practices (with a few affirmations to support you). If you feel those first flutterings of a flare, it is time to put your phone down and stop the busy headlong rush into your day – and learn the power of being present. Creating a place of presence, a sphere of stillness in your day, however small, however humble, will start you on the journey home to your gut. And remember, if you think you don't have time and you are too busy for even a few minutes, then your flare may build – because the body keeps the score. Your flare is a message to you from your gut – it's time to listen.

### Flare reflection

Get your Gut-loving Journal and take a few moments. In the most loving way you can, ask yourself the following questions. I suggest asking them out loud and then writing down your answers.

- What is causing me anxiety or overthinking?
- Have I taken on too much?
- Where in my life am I overcommitted?
- Who can support me?
- What can I do today to let go, simplify and surrender?
- How do I feel about the next week, month?

As you write, drop any temptation to judge yourself.

When you do these oh-so simple, so beautiful bits of inner work, you create a compassionate space for you and your dear gut.

### *Affirmations and mindfulness practice*

Stress creeps up on us. It accumulates slowly, drop by drop until we overflow. When you flare, try not to get frustrated with yourself or your gut. I know that can be hard if that's your habit. Instead, send love to any part of your body having a hard time.

What do you need most when you're feeling sore? I'm guessing not a telling-off or a cold shoulder. We need love, clear and simple. To be heard. To be understood. Language is powerful. How you direct your energy and thoughts is powerful. So try loving that gorgeous gut of yours.

Mindfulness has so many health benefits, but in practice, it can feel like we are pushing against a whole society of busyness. So how can you create a simple sphere of awareness in your day? Well, I want to share with you – it can be so easy.

Take affirmations. They can be wonderful ways to raise awareness of those parts of your body which deserve to be celebrated, not ignored. Affirmations can be a tool. I suggest using the Belly Metta Bhavana practice *(page 79)* as the basis of freestyling and creating the perfect words of healing and support for yourself. What is it you need to hear and affirm?

## Breathe out gut-loving affirmations

Here are a few affirmations that you can use daily, whenever it feels right for you, to offer your gut some love:

- I love my colon. I care for my ileum.
- I cherish my beloved gut bugs.

You can even focus on those you feel you need to nurture.

- I love my lactobacillus – thank you.
- My beautiful plicae circulares, thank you.
- My precious ileum, I send you loving light.

Deepen your affirmations further by saying them while looking in the mirror, into your eyes. Or record them on your phone and play them back when you need to deepen your self-care. Keep smiling as you think of all those lovelies in your gut working hard to keep a balance in your core – all that lives within you.

## *Begin with your breath*

If you're new to mindfulness – or maybe you've tried and failed to keep a regular mindfulness practice – you might ask, where do I begin?

The simple answer is you begin with the breath. So today, start to commit to daily mindfulness practice. However small, however humble (start with three minutes), this is the thread that will start to bridge the disconnect between you and your gut. Mindfulness is about learning to show up for yourself. It really is that simple.

There is a little bit of a tendency to believe that mindfulness practice, like meditation, might need to involve a special cushion, sitting cross-legged, and maybe a gong. Having used all those things, they are lovely parts of a ritual for coming home to yourself. But all you really need is your breath. And the good news is that you have that all the time. So let's have a go together right now.

## Mindful gut-care practice

For this exercise, I don't recommend lying down but sitting in an open, alert, but fully relaxed way.

1. Notice how you're sitting. The main point is to have a straight back and a stable posture. You may feel drawn to cross your legs. If it's comfortable, go for it, but if you're twisting yourself into a leg knot – drop that and sit in a chair with your feet firmly on the ground.

2. Now notice your chest and your belly and see if you can feel them in an open and relaxed way. As you do so, you'll automatically notice your spine lengthens. There's a slight natural curve to your neck, so that might mean your chin is a tiny bit tucked in. In the Buddhist tradition in which I trained, I was taught to leave the mouth slightly open and eyes open but soft and natural. If leaving your eyes open is too distracting, then it's fine to close your eyes, too, especially if you are new to mindfulness.

3. So spend a minute shuffling around a little – and getting really comfortable in your body and your position.

4. Once you're comfy, open and relaxed, you very naturally start to notice your breath. Don't try and change it. Just notice it. It's particularly helpful to notice your out-breath. What's interesting is, as you start to become aware of your exhale, it naturally starts to deepen and slow a little. You may even feel drawn to taking a few deep breaths. Go with that.

OK, you are practising mindfulness right now. What you'll spot is that your mind may start to fill with thoughts, like I've got to go and get dinner on. Is that the sound of a car alarm? And well, the practice is just to notice them. Don't try to stop them. Just notice them gently. 'OK, I've gone off... I'm thinking,' as soon you spot this, gently bring yourself back to noticing your breath. Thoughts will pop up, and that's fine. Thoughts will come and go. That's fine, just notice them, like a passer-by – but don't follow them down the street.

If you're new to mindfulness, just aim for three or five minutes. Yep, just a few moments and then go on back into your day. What I do recommend is to aim to do this several times a day. What you'll notice is that if you do this, say, four or five times a day, you'll naturally start to notice times when you just come back to your breath in a really relaxed, more aware state.

That, dear one, is the whole point of mindfulness practice. The more you do it, the more you start to just notice when you've rushed off into busy. You'll notice that busy is still there, but you'll spot the overthinking, stressed-out mind a little earlier, and you'll start to notice a little more space around the busy. Because you've got this lovely, super simple tool that you can use anytime, in any situation. As Eckhart Tolle reminds us: 'Rather than being your thoughts and emotions – be the awareness behind them.'

A great comparison for what you are doing – either as someone new to mindfulness or an experienced meditator – is it's a little like doing free weights at the gym. You don't start with the 50kg (110lbs), which might just overwhelm and strain your muscles. You start with little weights, the 5kg (11lbs) and build up slowly. Crucially you celebrate the fact that you've just turned up and remembered. What I know for sure is that as you become more aware of your breath, slowly, slowly, your head, heart and gut will start to align in your daily life. You will be more self-aware, less likely to overextend yourself.

*The act of mindfulness is just about the most caring, compassionate thing you can do for yourself.*

### *Building micro-moments of mindfulness into your day*

Today have a go at finding those micro-moments. Right now, think of ways to be creative in how you **remember to remember**. When you pop the kettle on, take a breath. When you flip on your laptop, take a breath. When you hear a ping from your phone – yeah, what a great little regular reminder that one is – take a breath. And what about those minor irritations? Can you turn those into little nudges to remember a mindful breath: waiting in a queue, a traffic light? All these are great opportunities. Before you eat – and yes, you know the biology of setting up your dear digestive tract for success – try taking three mindful breaths. Aim to thread a strong yet gentle thread of awareness of your breath into your day. Yes, as you dot your day with these glimpses of space, you'll notice you feel a greater sense of calm and ease, and your gut will be oh-so grateful.

- **Seek the calm centre of your life by simplifying.** There is nothing like being ill to focus you on what really matters. Take stock – knowing stressful life events can trigger a flare. What's going on for you right now?

- **Don't underestimate the power of stress.** It's not just all in the mind. Monday mornings are the time people are most likely to have a heart attack.[25] We are hard-wired to respond with powerful physiological responses to cortisol and adrenaline. We are embodied, and we know self-compassion can reduce inflammation in our bodies.

- **Try little and often.** So keep building those compassionate, mindful moments in your day and rest in them. Trust you are starting your healing journey. I know it can be hard to do, especially if you are in flare; then your painful bloated belly needs calm. Keep breathing into it; keep on listening like your life depends on it!

- One of the reasons that we focus on developing mindfulness and compassion practices is to **prepare for the tough times in life**. Gently remind yourself that everyone, I mean everyone, goes through tough times – even those who look like their lives are perfect. Socially prescribed perfectionism has gone crazy – yes, we're all so busy worrying and comparing ourselves to filtered selfies that we squeeze out the inner voice. We are at risk of assuming that everyone has 'all their shit together', and hey, you know the truth.

## ♥ Gut Love ♥

Use this **bloat action plan** to help you find comfort when you need it.

- Breathe deeply. It stimulates your vagus nerve, and can support your digestive reset and get you tuned in to your parasympathetic system.
- Get outside and go for a walk – keep it gentle.
- Try not to go to bed bloated. Instead, try gentle stretching to stimulate gut motility
- Drink fresh peppermint tea. Steep a few home-grown sprigs of this easy-growing herb in hot water and sip slowly.
- Chew fennel seeds.
- Give yourself permission to put your health before everything else. Your job, your studies, your relationship. Yep, for a few weeks, just make yourself and your gut a priority. If that makes you feel guilty, then get some coaching or some counselling to explore that.

## *The transformative power of journalling*

Your gut counts; it is a precious piece of kit. And if it's not working right, then nothing in your life will be quite right. When you arrive on the other side of your flare/bloat (and you will), build in some time to reflect. Take stock of the flare when you are ready to. When you are feeling strong, ask yourself *What just happened?* Be curious, compassionately curious. And please remember to try not to beat yourself up. That will just get you stuck where you are, and you want to move forwards. Treat your body and your gut like the wondrous inner world they are. You are the curator of your gut, the tender carer of that world.

If you are in the headspace to manage to look both ways in your life, then do it. What's just been happening with you? What have you been eating? How have you been eating? What's been going on in your life? Can you see a trigger? Or is it a combination of factors?

If there's nothing obvious to you, or it feels just too complicated, then invite a friend or trusted gut gang member to spend some time with you. Good listening can support you in unravelling the situation. If there's real trauma in your life, work or relationships, get the expert support you need. Reach out. There are so many organizations that can offer support – I've made a list for you of my top picks in the Resources section. Now, we know our illness sits in the midpoint between the stuff we can't control (the past, our unique recipe book of DNA), but we also have the writing in the margins of our very own cookbook, and we can spice up our recipes, swap out old ingredients and make our own healing choices. Because whatever our background, our history and our heritage, we get to decide today on the choices we make right here, now.

Illness can be heavy work. Even in its midst, there's a chance to seek out a deeper relationship with ourselves. Inspired by her time as a palliative carer, Bronnie Ware wrote about the top five regrets of the dying,[26] and number one was: 'I wish I'd had the courage to live a life true to myself, not the life others expected of me.'

Being honest about what's going on with ourselves and others – we get permission to show up authentically – just as we are.

## Talking to your partner

In a relationship, share as much or as little as you feel comfortable with. It is best to have a chat about your gut health issues when you're well and let your partner (old or new) know your symptoms and how you manage them.

Choose a time when you can talk honestly, openly and calmly. Maybe over dinner – that will feel like a natural time to chat – especially if your food choices are a little unusual or there's food (on the menu or on the table) you know doesn't sit well with your gut. If it's a new relationship, you might want to go easy on some of the details – keep it light, and of course, a little humour about your poop habits goes a long way. But make sure if you do that, you leave the conversation open so you can go back to it and tell them more another time.

For new or old relationships, actually letting your partner know what you need to heal and recover is a bit of a gift for your relationship. So be brave and tell them what it's like for you. I'd recommend just noticing how your partner shows up for you in your flare and fear. If you're anything like me, you'll probably not want to make too much of a fuss, and you might not want to bother others. But being honest helps deepen your connection. In fact, there's increasing evidence that isolation and loneliness are bad for our health and for our gut diversity. As Dilip. V. Jeste MD, Distinguished Professor of Psychiatry and Neurosciences at UC San Diego School of Medicine, states:

> *Lower levels of loneliness and higher levels of wisdom, compassion, social support and engagement were associated with greater phylogenetic richness and diversity of the gut microbiome.*[27]

If you're not in a relationship, then chat to friends and family, and of course, follow your gut. I've known some folk to be fully open with everyone, and others go a little more slowly with even close family. Be brave, take it slow, but keep having those gut-loving conversations.

Honestly, pretty much everyone has gut health issues at some point – gut health matters, even for those folks with apparently healthy guts. Colon cancer is a killer. By being open, you just might open up a conversation that saves someone else's life. Yes, really. Don't' be afraid to be clear on what you need to live your best gut life. Being open is actually about self-care and self-compassion, and done in the right way, it may be a crucial element of your healing. Sometimes during a flare, you can feel alone. Having some support from friends, family and your partner is all about gut-loving support – the best kind.

## Gut reflecting

Take out your Gut-loving Journal and ask yourself the following questions.

- What gives you joy? If in doubt – do that. Or a version of that joy that is possible in your flare. Keep it simple. We have a knack for making our lives complicated.
- What gives you meaning? How can you bring more of this to your day, or your week, or take a long view this year?
- Who do you enjoy being around? Those members of your life team with no judgement. OK, hang out with them, doing all of the stuff above.

If you can play – yes, play. OK, you're thinking this is a book about loving and calming your gut, but it is also about tuning in to yourself – the whole of you. The sad stuff and mad stuff, and we're complicated. Even if you're flaring and bloated, you can have fun. The world doesn't need to stop. So drop the busy for a bit. Luxuriate in doing stuff that makes you smile – that has no other purpose than being those things that make you laugh.

## Above all, be kind

When we are in pain, our natural instinct is to fold inwards and down over the tender areas of our belly, but if you open out gently and kindly and breathe into the pain, you may find some relief. Much of our experience of pain is the actual closing/straining against our feelings. It's all this extra holding and shallow breathing that makes our pain feel like a weight in our body. Breathe in and relax into the pain.

If your bloating is painful, breathe into it and use gentle yoga and tai chi exercises (*see page 167*) to massage and care for your gut. Above all, be **the right kind of gentle for you**. Sometimes when we are most anxious and afraid, we just have to let go and dance with our emotions. I'm going to share a secret about how I do that in Chapter 13.

## Stubborn flare – let's go a little deeper

Flaring can fill us with fear. Fear of what we can't see. Our flare can be triggered by stress – a little flicker – and then flare itself creates a cycle of worry that can increase our flare – until we have a whole forest fire burning in our gut.

If you're in a stubborn flare, do the practical stuff – work with your IBD or IBS team. Take the meds. Medication may dull or neutralize the pain of IBD or IBS (and some meds can be vital in the healing journey), but intuition tells us that deeper healing takes place only when we heed the energy that sits behind the pain.

Many of us experience our lives against a diffuse background of low-level stress. We may feel overwhelmed. Overwhelm equals disconnect – from ourselves and our anxious, irritable and inflamed gut. As cortisol rises, we feel stress and anxiety. Our language speaks this 'gut-wrenching' truth. Suffering contracts us. We close down, our bellies harden, our guts inflame. So how do you honour the feelings of fear and anxiety? How do you offer them space to be acknowledged beyond the tight ridges of our intestinal wall?

The experience of stress sits deep in the core of our being. Through visualizations, we may discover traumatic and stressful experiences held in our gut. As we deepen our inward self-compassion journey, we start to untangle these energetic roots in our belly. For me, these strands of shock and trauma have hardened in my gut. The roots took hold when I felt most vulnerable – the points in my own life experience when I felt metaphorically punched in the gut.

Trauma sits in our bodies, and it holds a resonance. Body and breathwork can be powerful techniques to gently enter into these stuck places. We can start slowly to do this inner process independently or may need the support of a therapist or healer. When you go deeper into your own stories, you may even find some of them are not your own. You may well find older family patterns of pain, trapped and repeated. These deeper energetic patterns of emotion and stuck energy hang around in our guts.

Gut healing work takes us deeper into the solar plexus chakra, which sits in the upper belly and is associated with personal power and identity (*see figure 4, page 30*). In this way, our gut health troubles can be seen as a way of working more deeply with how we show up in the world and an opportunity to express ourselves authentically. Blocked or repressed energy asks us to go deeper into our life purpose and our longing to show our true self.

Through deepening your mindfulness practice and belly breathwork, you nourish this chakra. As you continue to start to grow your self-awareness, you may start to notice the ways that your gut instincts want to guide you to be truer to yourself in your day-to-day interactions and life choices.

My own gut trouble revealed a deep disconnect between the pressures I felt to succeed and how I wanted to live my life. As you start to go deeper into your intuitive breathwork, visualizations and affirmations in this book, you may find that you start cultivating a relationship where you learn to trust and follow your gut.

## Gut-healing visualization

This exercise is best done with your eyes closed, lying flat on your back, palms open at your sides.

1. Breathe deeply down into your root chakra (*see figure 4, page 30*). As you do this, imagine holding a little of your breath on your exhale in the root chakra. Do this three times, and then just release the breath in a slow, gentle exhale. This will ground your energy in a deep and nourishing way and awaken your awareness of the energetic flow of your chakras.

2. Slowly turn your attention to your solar plexus chakra. Depending on your sensory tendency, you may feel a subtle swirling, a little like water going down a plughole. Or you might get a visual sense of colour. This chakra is associated with the amber spectrum of light.

3. Stay here for a little, breathing into this chakra and feeling the energy. If you have pain or discomfort, gently, lovingly breathe into that pain. Suspend judgement and just feel the energy of that pain. Is it moving at a higher or lower vibration than the rest of your body? Is it hot, hard, heavy, dull? Keep breathing into and feeling it. You may get a strong visual sense of it. How does the pain look? What colour is it?

4. What you'll notice is that pain is just energy, held or blocked. Keep noticing and feeling. Bring your attention to this chakra. If you feel your focus shift up or down your body, go with this. The chakras are

interconnected (like pearls on a string), so you may notice areas of energy withdrawal. You may feel a release of energy.

5. After a few minutes, place your open palms on your belly. As you do this, visualize love and light going into your solar plexus chakra. Trust that this light is nourishing and healing your colon, your ileum and all the delicate organs of digestion at a deeper energetic level.

6. When you are ready, return to your breath and your day. Repeat when you feel the need to go deeper.

To extend and deepen this practice, complete three breaths into each of your chakras, focusing, in particular, on the flow of energy between the sacral and heart chakras, which link directly to your solar plexus chakra.

---

Follow your gut wisdom. Simply breathing deeply can start to unlock the stuck places and connect your gut, your heart and your head in a fresh way – towards a deeper alignment with your being. In my own gut journey, I have found this exercise is a powerful tool to energize and align all the chakras. Breathe with heartfelt compassion to your gut.

## The deep work

Sometimes we feel things are so fixed, so stuck. The reality is that like wind on water, our emotions shift and change. We feel where energy and emotion have got trapped or contracted. We unknot and untangle. Sometimes it'll happen suddenly, a rich buzz of intense emotion and release – stuck energy releases in vibration, heat and breath, and sometimes movement. In Chapter 13, we'll explore the power of dance to release and transmute unexpressed anger and shame into a fluid flow of energy.

Once you uncover the root of your gut pain, you can start to unravel the knots of your gut narrative. At this stage, you begin to heal. Through gut knowledge and gut compassion, you naturally find the deeper motivation to self-care and gut care, but without the inner work, you may end up playing on the surface.

*Tough love just leaves us shifting the furniture of our lives, not moving to our true home. Telling yourself off only gives power to the voice of your inner critic.*

Without the inner work, you may find that you take on a punishing elimination diet or fitness regime. It may even work for a while. But it's not true healing. The deeper healing begins when you unravel the knots, soften the light and start to witness all the ways your body needs to be heard and understood. If you feel drawn to the deep work, then I recommend reading the work of two leading thinkers on the work of self-compassion: Tara Brach and Kristin Neff. It is beyond this book's scope to go deeply into our inner repressed emotions, but when you complete these exercises it's highly likely you'll uncover further work to do. So I share further resources, especially on deepening self-compassion, at the back of this book (*see page 262*).

## Chapter 12

# Movement and Microbiome

*'If you just set people in motion, they'll heal themselves.'*

Gabrielle Roth[28]

Movement helps us to heal. Our bodies want to be whole; it takes a lot of energy to stay stuck in the hard places of our bellies. Trust that your wisdom will take you to the right places. *Calm Your Gut* is a stepping-stone on the path of your healing journey. Step lightly and rest for a while before choosing your next step to good gut health. When things are uncertain, we need to be agile. We only have to look back at the start of 2020 – a year when unexpected global change shook us all up, to see that we live in fluid times. When we feel more flexible in our bodies, we have greater resilience in our minds. Flexible thinking enables us to respond from a place of *choice* rather than *fear*.

There's a risk when we talk about exercise that it's just another way of beating up our body and our gut. Being tough on yourself with punishing routines and unsustainable gym schedules isn't gut healing. Does your exercise regime, or lack of it, form a key backdrop to your negative self-talk? Do you feel like you're doing too little or too much? We all have stories about the right amount and what we should be doing.

What we do know is that movement is protective for gut health. Exercise has anti-inflammatory effects. People with IBD and IBS who are physically active have fewer flares and less serious outcomes than those who don't.[29] Exercise is also linked to a reduced risk of colon cancer.[30] It's also worth considering that some of the common anti-inflammatory meds used to treat IBD can interfere with bone-building cells – meaning a potential increase in the risk of fractures. So if you've been taking meds for a few years, you need to strengthen your bones with weight-bearing exercises like dance, running or weights.

But before you sign up for a marathon, there's evidence that excessive exercise can trigger digestive distress. Even folk with healthy guts can suffer from runner's trot. A flare and an intense workout may just be all too much. Whatever you do, you need to firstly check in with your body and your gut. Find your own way into the stuff you love; the stuff that gives you joy, that connects you to your body. The body is the mind.

*Right now, today – how can you honour your body's need for movement?*

## Yoga is not just exercise

There's an ancient wisdom tradition at the root of yoga. Yoga has been shown to reduce stress, and inflammation, relieving symptoms in both ulcerative colitis and IBS.[31] Yoga is a sequence of movements to stretch out the stuck places in our bodies – a way to connect our body with its own wisdom. We see it in animals: the delicate post-snooze stretch of your cat, the playful downward dog of a pup. When you spend more time in movement, you'll be amazed how quickly your body starts to show you how it wants to move in the world. How it needs to be to create a more balanced belly and biome.

Yoga poses which stretch and energize the root chakra (*see figure 4, page 30*) tend to focus on the softening of the abdominal area through core body twists and deep diaphragmatic breathing. Yoga poses with mindful breathing help release any tension we hold at our core. This is where we have found the language of the anxious gut, the hard, swollen gut.

*Yoga is one of the most gut-loving ways to start your day.*

Yoga can also be a great way of toning your muscles and keeping the pelvic floor strong. A weak pelvic floor and lower digestive tract can be caused by poor pooping technique or repeated visits to the toilet. There's some evidence that those of us with IBD and IBS need to take extra care of our pelvic floor. When toned and activated, this group of muscles between the tailbone and the pubic bone supports gut health. You might also want to invest in a poop stool. Our bodies and digestive tract were designed to squat, not sit. Squatting is a much more efficient way to release our bowels and creates less strain. Daily gentle yoga practices can provide restorative gut care.

## Yoga poses to heal

You'll need a good yoga mat or a folded blanket in a large rectangle on a non-slippery floor. Have bare feet and loose clothing. What you wear needs to enable deep breathing and ease of movement for your belly and lower back. If you're new to yoga, listen to your body, and go gentle and slow on your joints and spine.

## Reclining twist

Use this pose to release any pent-up feelings in your belly area and support vagal stimulation. Combine the pose with deep breaths to connect to your beloved gut.

1. Lie on your back with arms outstretched either side and palms facing upwards.
2. Bend your right knee and place your right foot on your left knee.
3. As you exhale, drop your right knee over to the left side of your body, twisting your spine and lower back.
4. Rest in this position, aiming to keep your shoulders flat to your mat. Look along your right arm to your fingertips.
5. As you breathe, let gravity pull your knee to the floor. Be gentle and ease out of the movement slowly.
6. To release, inhale and roll your hips back into the front and as you exhale, lower your right leg back to the mat.

## Cat/cow

I shared this pose earlier in the book (*see page 101*), but cat/cow is also a great way to tone and move your lower back and the abdominal area. This pose can shape more mindful breathing into the base of the belly, gently massaging your gut. It also enables a shifting and release of energy in the lower chakras.

## Warrior pose II

This is a pose of strength and balance. Perfect for our fiercely compassionate approach to our gut health. You will need to be super stable on the floor (ditch the blanket) and stand on a hard surface. To deepen the grounding presence of this pose, do it outside on the earth or grass.

1. Step outwards with your right foot in front, toes forwards, and your left foot behind with your toes aligning parallel to your mat.

2. Now bend your right knee, so it is directly over your ankle, and try to balance your weight across both feet.

3. Now shift your shoulders so that you face outwards over your body and lift your straight arms outwards, palms facing down as though you are a tight-rope walker.

4. Rest in this posture, keeping your gaze in front of you, and breathe. Now turn and gaze along the line of your arm to your right fingertips and breathe deep into your belly for a cycle of seven breaths.

5. Now slowly inhale and straighten your right leg, and release.

6. Repeat on your left side.

## Knees to chest

This is a great pose if you are bloated and enables a gentle massage of the gut area. Be mindful where you do this one if you're super bloated!

1. Lie on your back with your knees bent and feet flat on the floor. Relax and breathe deeply here for a cycle of three in-out breaths. Aim to ease your lower back and neck onto the mat in a relaxed position so you feel stable and held.

2. Now slowly bring each knee up towards your chest and hold them close together by wrapping your arms around your lower legs. If you can, loosely clasp the opposite arm to hold your position, but move in a way that's natural to your body. If this is uncomfortable, ease your knees apart and loosen the hold of your arms to enable your breath. Keep your neck and lower back pressed into the floor.

3. Relax, feel your spine held by the mat and breathe for at least seven deep belly breaths into your solar plexus and root chakra (*see*

*page 30*). When you are ready, slowly release your arms and return your feet to the ground one at a time.

4. If you are comfortable in this position, you can extend it by very gently rocking from side to side, the slightest subtle movement.

## Child's pose

Resting in **child's pose** is a lovely way of curving into the belly and protecting it. This pose can stimulate the vagus nerve and support a deep sense of peace. Hence it is a safe place to return to during your yoga routine, somewhere you may instinctively return to during a gut flare.

1. Kneel on all fours on your yoga mat. Keep your knees open with big toes touching, and hands the width of your yoga mat apart. Inhale.
2. As you exhale, lean your body between your knees, and reach your arms out flat in front of you with your palms facing down.
3. The aim is to touch your forehead to the floor. If there is any strain in this, have an extra folded blanket ready to support your head and raise it off the floor.
4. As you rest in this position, relax your shoulders and your jaw. Just rest and restore.

For more support, try the gentle and inspiring sequences by Adriene at www.yogawithadriene.com.

*Move with self-care at*
*the core of what you do.*

## Mindful movement

The synchronization of breath and movement naturally raises our awareness and our connection to the present moment. I also love the magical feel of qigong, stillness and flowing movement. Qigong harmonizes and strengthens by increasing energy flow throughout the body, creating a sense of calm. Moving mindfully through space is the heart of these spiritual practices and building this foundation into your day or your week can extend to greater awareness in your life.

When we start to integrate even a few moments of mindfulness into our day, we find ourselves becoming more present. In Buddhism, there is an expression called the 'view'. It's a space of wakeful presence, which we start to establish through regular meditation practice. The purpose of mindfulness is to retain the 'view' in action. **How do we retain a more awake perspective even in the doing of our lives?**

Qigong, yoga and tai chi, like all energetic activity exercises, are about restoring balance, practising awareness and being more present to ourselves. They are ways to practise being present whilst moving. These are practices of gut care and self-compassion. As always, go with your gut and find the practice that works for you.

Some go-to gut-loving exercises include:

- **Cycling** is a lovely gentle mindful exercise. No pollution, just presence.
- **Walking** – you would be forgiven for forgetting that walking is our natural state, not sitting. There is so much evidence of the health benefits of standing and walking during our day. If you feel energetic, **running is fun and free**.
- **Tree dancing** is best on a windy day. Want to connect with your inner wild woman or man? Find a group of trees and simply attune to their movement. Barefoot is best. Sway to the trees'

rhythm, and you'll feel a deeply grounded connection to the natural world.

- **Gardening** is earthy mindfulness. And you can produce seasonal home-grown organic food for your gut. #breatheyourmicrobiome

Now to one of my favourite fun ways of connecting heart, mind and gut through dance.

## Chapter 13

# GUT HEALING DANCE

*'When did you stop dancing? When did you stop singing? ... When did you stop being comforted by the sweet territory of silence?'*

Gabrielle Roth, dancer and urban shaman

In or out of a flare, building gentle and restorative movement into your day or week can help heal. As you start to explore your own journey of healing into your belly, you may find old patterns of holding in the area of your root chakra (*see figure 4, page 30*).

Intuitive movement can unlock the stuck places of the body. It can help release the flow of energy, from the sacral chakra to the solar plexus chakra and then to the heart. Through yoga, deep breathing and dance, we get the chance to release and unknot the kinks of our colon and the tight holding places of our anxious gut. In this space, energy work, breathwork and dance are a powerful trio.

So much of adulting is an endless rinse and repeat. We tend to follow the same old ruts of habit, good or bad, over and over. When you dance with the intention of connecting to your gut, you can innocently get deep into your body and be childlike again. You tune in to your body with your own gut-led authentic movement.

In the liminal space of dance, we have the opportunity to let go, to learn new steps. We may start to unravel the knots of countless commutes and tense team meetings – the stuff we don't say. The stuff that kinda gets set in our body and our gut. You know the places in your body where you are tight. Our own armoury is so familiar we may have stopped feeling it. It's easier to see in others – the tight neck, the crease between the brow, the uneven shape of shoulders. Dance can be a way of loosening the habit knots. As we dance, we start to align our chakras.

## The Gut Love Dance

This dance is inspired by the work of Gabrielle Roth and the ancient Maori haka. The haka is a potent display of intention, somewhere between a dance and a ritual of battle. I have a deep respect and love for this ritual. Gabrielle Roth's own work was in part inspired by Carl Jung's study of the collective unconscious mind and how the stories we tell ourselves shape our world view.

When we are ill, we can feel like the victim. Dance is a creative and expansive way of opening up how we relate to ourselves and our sense of personal agency and integrity. Integrity, like self-compassion, can have an edge of steel – a fierce determination. **The Gut Love Dance** is a way to ignite your breath, energize your body and inspire your **spirit** – just what you most need when you feel vulnerable and disconnected. When we sit in a blurred busyness of poor health and stress, sometimes we cannot envision a way out.

Dance is emotion embodied in action. When the juncture between **who** I am and **how** I am has become too large – just when my sore and swollen guts need to be restored – I dance. For many of us, the experience of getting ill is an experience of disconnect: 'The dance is not where we lose ourselves, but where we find ourselves.'[32]

## Gut Love Dance

Start by creating a mindful environment. Find a space for your Gut Love Dance. To be free to experiment, I suggest you start your first one alone. Choose music to inspire strength and freedom

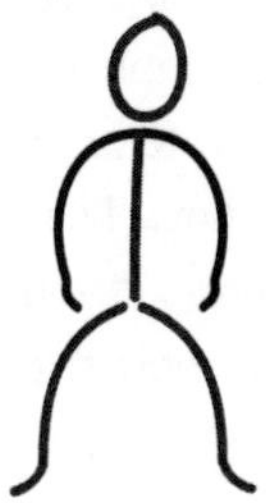

1. Stand with your feet a little wider apart than your shoulders with your knees slightly bent in a relaxed, open stance. Keep your hands loose at your sides with palms facing inwards. Breathe. See if you can almost sit very slightly into this posture. In tai chi and qigong, this position is a dynamic starting point.

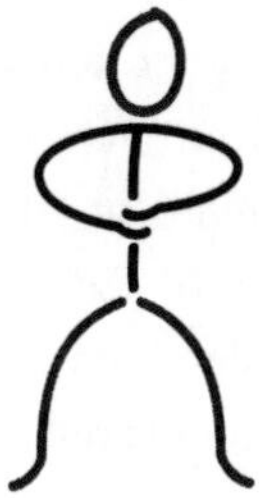

2. Place your palms at the base of your belly and breathe into this for three breaths. As you breathe out, make a loud, audible sigh 'ahhh'. Let the volume build each time you exhale. From this position, form fists and fold your arms across your solar plexus; this is your base position. You will return to this during your Gut Love Dance.

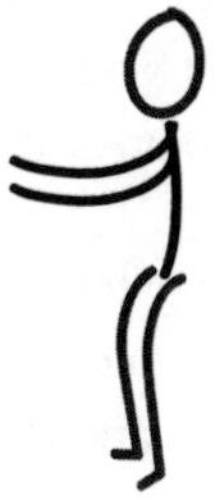

3. Now lower your arms, and then slowly draw your hands upwards along the midline of your body (breathing inwards deeply). As you draw your hands upwards, stop at each of the key chakra points and push outwards. Release your fists so that your palms are open and exhale as you push outwards away from your sacral chakra, your solar plexus chakra, your heart and throat chakras.

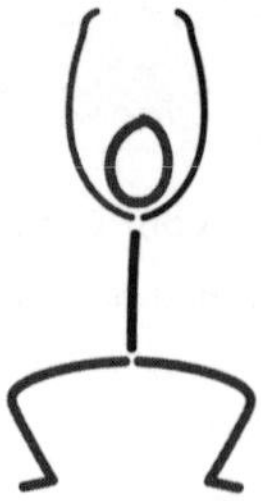

4. Repeat this cycle – alternating pushing your palms out from your throat, heart and belly, exhaling loudly as your hands move out. As you push out from your belly area, think of what you need to release. What is stuck? What needs to go? To deepen your breath, you can sway your belly back and forth as you breathe. From your throat, what do you need to say? Keep it simple – you may find a word or phrase repeating. Go with it. The Gut Love Dance is about connecting to your body, so if you find yourself getting too caught in words, come back to the breath.

   After a few minutes, your breathing will have deepened. Now move your arms up and outwards to embody your fierce gut compassion. Hold a 'strong man' or 'strong woman' pose and deepen this by extending your legs outwards and sinking into them. Smile to yourself and your gorgeous gut.

   Take your fists back to your belly. Feel your strength and compassion. Hold this movement. This is your Gut Love Dance – let it be a dance of intention. Healing, strength, compassion.

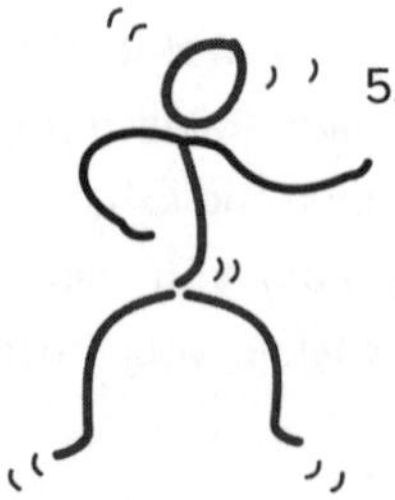

5. Now let's get playful and creative; this is your safe space to move as your body and your gut need. The right music can inspire and liberate you! Move into your hips and shoulders and sway slowly, loosening up. This is the time to fully engage your belly in your dance.

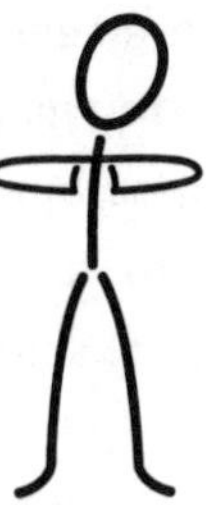

6. When you feel it is time, breathe into your fear, your frustration, your rage, your anxiety – give them shape. If you are in a flare, give it a shape, a movement. You may even find that you need to dance to honour your ancestors. Those who came first, before you in the gut journey. Those who raised your grandparents and parents to this life. If it feels right, dance as an offering to them. Find a place to let go of any unfinished emotion; dance it out and come back to it as you feel. And breathe. Dance to your gut, your heart and your head. Trust the inner work to happen. It will.

   When your dance feels complete, slow gradually and come back to your breath. When you are ready, hold your hands with palms facing your chest and bow deeply to yourself and your gut for honouring your need to move.

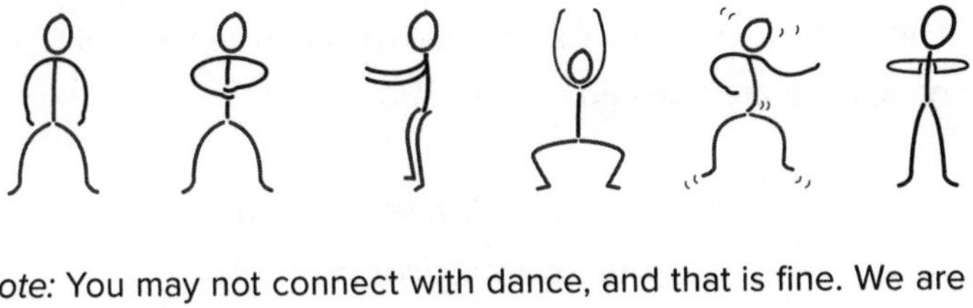

*Note:* You may not connect with dance, and that is fine. We are all embodied in different ways. If, however, you find that you are stuck in your head, don't underestimate the chance to connect with your heart and gut. Music can really help with this. Choose something that will free you to connect more to yourself and move.

*We dance to reconnect to our body and our gut.*

Our bodies hold memories in our muscles, and movement goes deeper than words. Bodywork like this is powerful. You may find deep emotions are released or shifted. Trust the process, but if you feel stuck in your emotions after three or four sessions, it may be time to seek help from a coach, counsellor or therapist to share the processing of your emotions.

My first gut dance was born out of my own experience of feeling frustrated and down about being bloated. I had experienced a mini flare. Overworked and out of balance, it was a time I needed to dig deep and recommit to myself. I felt the need to recommit symbolically to both my beloved gut and to the hard-won knowledge of my elimination diet – a time to bring body and spirit into alignment.

Amid the movements, we align our intention with action. Dance can transmute energy. The Gut Love Dance can act as a bridge to gut integrity – honouring our whole being. When we are no longer at war with our bodies, we show a deep commitment to listening and taking care of them. That process will require, at times, fearless and fierce compassion. We may have to face shame or embarrassment about aspects of our lives and ways of living. Create your own Gut Love Dance – the key is to channel whatever emotions you feel right now into its creation. You may even want to connect with your gut gang to create a shared dance.

*In the Gut Love Dance, you stand*
*your sacred ground.*

### *Dance to align head, heart and gut*

During your Gut Love Dance, you can chant affirmations or even just keywords like strength, healing, compassion – as this stimulates the vagus nerve. However you engage with dance, it will ground your body into your breath, and your breath into your gut, and into alignment with yourself.

We know that too often in the language of medicine, we are seen to be at war with our bodies, battling the parts of ourselves that have failed us; for those of us with IBD and IBS, those parts of our guts that we believe have let us down. Here at the point of gut healing, we are moving TOWARDS GUT INTEGRITY, so we reframe this relationship. The Gut Love Dance is part of both your healing and your integrity. It is something to take away and create. Be powerful and playful.

The dance is never *against* our gut. We never battle our bodies. How can we battle ourselves? Your intention at the close of your Gut Love Dance is a renewed commitment to your gut. To unite body, mind and spirit as one.

If you need the inspiration, you can do a shorter, essential gut dance in hospital toilets – a jolt of positivity before heading in for a blood test or colonoscopy. My own gut dance varies – sometimes fun, sometimes serious, sometimes strengthening.

### ♥ Gut Love ♥

Barefoot dancing on grass is particularly grounding for the anxious gut.

Let the dance meet you where you are and reset your Intention – purposeful self-care. Dance is a ritual beyond the limits of words, to the feelings beneath – a way to engage with your unconscious mind. As you develop gut knowledge and gut intelligence, dance can nourish the voice of your intuition, because your gut doesn't always need silence and space to speak to you. Early on, it often does, but as time goes on, your gut can be creative in communicating. Your Gut Love Dance can be two-way. To express the intention of fierce, compassionate commitment to your gut and an opportunity to hear your gut.

When we feel strong, we feel empowered. Empowered self-compassion has a strength and a harmony of flow that shapes our movement and creates a success cycle. We now understand the cycle of inflammation and all the risks that it can hold. Inflammation is a silent killer; it moves by stealth through the body, causing damage to joints and the intestinal wall; it flows through the body–brain axis and risks our mental wellbeing.

To start an anti-inflammatory diet that is bespoke to your body, and to design ways of moving that fit your body type and your needs, is a gift. A gift of self-love and self-care that will reinforce the cycle of successful self-compassion. Move in ways that give you joy. Move in ways that make you laugh and smile.

## Reflection time

Take out your Gut-loving Journal and ask yourself the following questions:

- Today how can I reconnect to my body through movement?
- What movement did I most love as a child? Sport, games, whatever it may be?
- How can I use movement to loosen my belly and play?

# GUT HEALING

Reflecting on the practices in this part of the book, take time to write your personal **Gut Manifesto.** So take out your **Gut-loving Journal** and choose a fresh page. You may want to include references to your aim to deindustrialize your gut or explore what movements you can commit to in your day and week. Once you've written down your manifesto, sign and date at the bottom of the page. You can choose to go a step further by typing this up, signing and framing it, sharing it with those who care about you and putting it somewhere you can see in your home. Or simply making it a screen saver on your phone!

- What can you do this week towards gut healing?
- Create your personal food map for gut health.
- What anti-inflammatory lifestyle changes can you make?
- What is your gut flare action plan?
- How will you incorporate mindfulness practice and gut healing visualization into your life?
- What mindful movements do you feel drawn to in order to heal your gut?

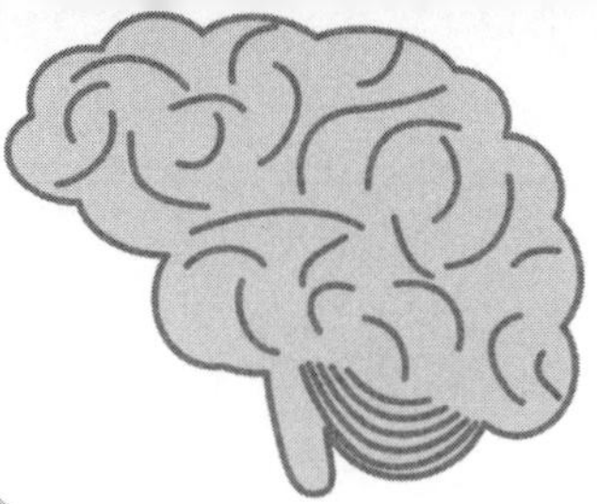

## Part IV

# GUT INTEGRITY

***'True happiness is when what you think, what you say and what you do are the same thing.'***

Mahatma Gandhi, Indian lawyer, politician, social activist and writer

As we heal, we grow our gut integrity.

Gut integrity is all about growing our gut resilience. We increase our gut integrity by consistently showing up for ourselves to create an anti-inflammatory lifestyle. We start to follow the call of our deeper intuitive gut. Over the following chapters, we're going to explore where we are right now as we stand at the crossroads of gut integrity.

We'll look at ways to become more gut articulate and connect with our wider gut gang. We'll keep reframing the gut narrative to get more gut empowered. While we do this, we'll keep returning to integrating sustainable change by building small hooks for new habits and celebrating our progress.

Connect to your gut wisdom and stay curious about what you can do to feel better.

## CHAPTER 14

# BECOMING GUT ARTICULATE

*'Your life depends on your power to master words.'*

ARTHUR SCARGILL, BRITISH TRADE UNIONIST

This area warrants a dedicated discussion at this stage in our gut healing journey. We've explored how becoming compassionately empowered leads to healing. So let's take another look at the 9m (29ft 6in) long tube of intelligent, sensitive biology, which houses 70 per cent of your immune system, processes food and enables life. This precious piece of kit influences how you feel, your energy levels and even your mental health. In fact, we can't be happy, whole human beings without a balanced biome. And one of the most important ways to support our gut journey is by becoming health articulate. This is my passion, and it's deeply personal.

I've seen so many folks struggle to navigate the health system and understand their own health. You know how it is. From busy GPs to overstretched NHS staff, too little time, so many sick people. This equation too often leads to a tendency to treat the *presenting* issue.

My dad got trapped in *prescription hazing*. I watched as the various parts of his body gave way – it was a slow incremental decline, and it started in his gut. Throughout his life, my dad suffered from crippling diverticulitis (gut inflammation). He had periods of debilitating insomnia due to the pain. He was of a generation and an era where his body was something that he just wanted to get on and do the job. You know the type; frustrated and let down when his body didn't obey his stubborn determination to keep going. His life was a lesson for me. Watching his fight with his body was a profound teaching because he never learned his body's language.

My dad couldn't enter into an equal dialogue with his doctor. It wasn't in his frame of reference. Doctors were respected and abided by – a generational attitude that's changing. We have more information, which gives us both greater agency and greater responsibility for our health. We are central to our own healing. As Jim Rohn[1] said, 'Take care of your body, it's the only place you've got to live.'

## Men and gut health

It's important to have an honest conversation about this, as traditionally men are less likely to visit their primary healthcare specialist and too often the treatment outcomes for men are a little poorer because of later diagnosis. We know this is a common gender difference across all illnesses. In some cases of IBD, this may increase the likelihood of later diagnosis[2] and potentially create complications. If you have a man in your life and something is not quite right, it's time to lovingly but firmly support them to access the expert treatment they deserve. Fierce compassion is both strong and loving.

There are also some clear differences in the experience of men and women with IBD. Concerning the gut gang, it's a big generalization, but women are more likely (but not always) to chat to others about their physical and mental wellbeing. It's exciting to see inspirational men leading the way to greater openness.

I am awed by the brave and honest men finding ways to articulate how they feel about their gut health and to express this through a range of forms.

When footballer Darren Fletcher spoke about living with ulcerative colitis, I know that many men with IBD connected to his story. He enabled them to share more with friends and family. Some inspirational men show it's possible to live a full life despite the challenges of IBD. Thank you, Olympic gold medallist Sir Steven Redgrave, rugby captain Lewis Moody, TV favourite Jeff Hordley, musician Dan Reynolds, NFL kicker Rolf Bernirschke and hockey pro Fernando Pisani, amongst many, many more. In my experience, men bring a particular kind of humour to the healing journey.

## Sharing your story

Ultimately, at this stage in your healing process, I hope you can embrace the courage and self-compassion to discuss what's going on with the people in your life. This is about owning your gut knowledge using the gut's language and getting to grips with the pain in a compassionately empowered way.

*Each time you speak, you are giving someone else permission to share their story.*

A key part of healing is learning your own health-articulate language. To be able to describe the discomfort in your descending colon. Where does it hurt, how does it hurt, when does it hurt? Once you have this, you will find that you can become more and more confident in communicating with the gut stakeholders in your life. So keep asking yourself:

- How willing am I to step up and be my own gut advocate?
- How willing am I to share my story with others and seek support to enable my journey towards my vision of gut integrity?

We can't talk about men without acknowledging that there are gender differences in gut health. Whilst IBD is relatively evenly distributed across men and women, IBS is overwhelmingly a female condition. This may in part be explained by underlying differences in the way the immune system responds in men and women. Also, by the additional reproductive organs[3] in our abdominal area – women have more kinks in their large intestine. Yes, women have literally got more curves on the inside too.

I'm grateful to the inspirational women who have shared their stories of living with IBD and flourishing despite the difficulty it can bring. A shout out to the wonderful women like professional dancer Amy Dowden, who shared her story in a BBC documentary, musician Anastacia, *Food Network* host Sunny Anderson, Olympic swimmer Siobhan-Marie O'Connor and *Made in Chelsea* star Louise Thompson, amongst so many others, for being out and proud and showing it is possible to thrive with IBD.

Men and women face different challenges with gut health, and women are more likely to report suffering from bloating and discomfort due to the menstrual cycle – this can exacerbate the symptoms of flare in Crohn's disease, ulcerative colitis and also IBS.[4] It's important to state that the sheer scale of the gender differences meant for many years the functional gut condition IBS was dismissed as being 'all in the head'. This links to a broader point about how we communicate and share how our gorgeous guts are doing, and more specifically how we go about communicating to the doctor in our lives.

The 'First Do No Harm' report into the NHS[5] by Baroness Julia Cumberlege talked of the deeply rooted 'defensiveness of the medical system' which in many significant ways remains hierarchical and male-orientated. Now that's a big generalization, and my gut instinct is that the situation is changing. What's fascinating about Cumberlege's report is the wider discussion around the culture of the medical profession. She felt that there remain some '... fundamental issues around power, justice, and compassion',[6] particularly when things don't go well.

I think part of the disconnect that can take place between patient and doctor is around language. If those of us with gut health issues are not fully articulate in navigating the system, then there's a risk that the patient's voice (non-expert) gets lost – that their voice has less weight, less value.

*We know that compassion is at the heart of the healing relationship with ourselves.*

Compassion's circle needs to embrace the relationship with our health professionals too. This type of honest compassion would enable a shared conversation about not just the symptoms but deeper causes. The process of becoming increasingly health and gut articulate places us in a position of greater equality. So how do we start to navigate the system to create a relationship based on equality and curiosity?

Undoubtedly there are many medical professionals, male and female, leading the way to rebalance the old hierarchy. The number of us with gut health issues is growing. This means there's a lot of money in the treatment protocols linked to the gut. There's a potentially darker side to the shape of the current medical system; there is a real risk that medical processes inadvertently service Big Pharma more than the individual patient. I don't believe that's a conscious process – I have met too many compassionate and caring doctors and medical professionals. What I do see is the surface-level treatment approach, maybe because the underlying causes are complex or simply endemic to modern city living.

Medicine can sometimes feel like a passive process. We let go of ourselves and our bodies to the medical protocol. In the arena of gut health, there is so much that is unique. An intricate combination of factors leads us to dis-ease. These factors take time to be unravelled. I speak as someone who is always deepening my own knowledge. And we know healing is not simply the event of popping a pill.

## Establishing a supportive gut gang

In an average 9–12-minute appointment with a GP, writing a prescription is easier than unravelling all the parts that might contribute to poor gut health. As we've discovered, when the gut is involved, it's complex, multifactorial and so often individualistic. What is exciting is that there is a new arena of 'lifestyle prescriptions' opening up a whole new dialogue with doctors. This is the start of a more interconnected perspective on the treatment of dis-ease.

Those of us with IBD and IBS are often the most health articulate, the most tuned in and switched on 'patients' on the planet, but it's not always the case. IBD is spreading, remember. In fact, it feels like we need to see our individual illness in that large circle of troubled guts globally. We are one of many. As you engage with equality with the medical professionals in your life and have more honest conversations about how you can play an empowered part in your gut health, you are, in your own way, supporting better gut treatment for everyone.

We are at a point in history where we have access to some incredible medical treatments. I am hugely grateful to intravenous steroids – they saved my life. I want to be clear on this. When I was lying in the hospital gravely ill, no positive visualizations or affirmations would fix me. No amount of celery juice or psyllium husk was going to sort out my gut right at that moment. No, I needed to respect the medical protocol provided by my expert consultant. I needed to follow the treatment plan. Toxic megacolon could have killed me or led to dramatic surgery.

Slowly, I was weaned from intravenous steroids to prednisolone tablets. I was lucky. The treatment bought me precious time to make sense and integrate the lessons that my illness had to teach me. I know that many of you with Crohn's disease and ulcerative colitis or IBS may have a different path, by choice or circumstance.

This decade will see the emergence of more sophisticated treatments. As our understanding of the microbiome becomes more personalized, we will have a beautifully unique prescription of bacteria to heal each gut. New treatments in gut health are emerging. For now, there is no shame in taking conventional medication – sometimes, that really is the only way to reduce the life-restricting symptoms. At times it's only when we make it to the other side of a medical crisis that we have the mental and physical resources to really start to consider the wider life changes we may need to make. That's OK too.

The heart of this book is about empowering a calming and compassionate relationship with your gut. From this compassionate stance, I'm holding a middle ground. All too often, the traditional, conventional medical establishment is set against alternative and complementary practice. I want to call that out – there's an artificial sense of division. There are profound, holistic wisdom traditions that sit outside of Western medical approaches. And one of the pitfalls of Western medicine is that the premium placed on medical specialism means there's a tendency to atomize the body into different parts rather than view it as a *whole*.

Studies on the placebo effect[7] give us a glimpse into the psychology of healing and, in particular, the importance of the 'healing relationship'. We know that being given space and time to express what's going on supports healing. So if you don't get the compassionate, healing relationship with your doctor, be brave and seek it out with others (in addition to your conventional treatment plan). Follow your own wisdom. Remember, you can be your own gut advocate.

## A calm colonoscopy

Right now, let's turn our attention to some of the practical procedures we almost certainly undergo with the medical professionals in our lives to get the right diagnosis.

Is it possible to have a calm colonoscopy?

Well, sure it is. Right now, if you're reading this book, you've probably been up close and personal with various camera investigations. Or maybe you are hoping for one or waiting for one. We know if we have IBD that we have an increased risk of developing colon cancer,[8] so having a regular scope is an important preventative measure to monitor your gut's health. Bowel cancer rates are on the up, and the number of young people with colon cancer has increased at a higher rate.[9] So let's get into the nitty-gritty of the whole thing because preparing for and undergoing a colonoscopy is not fun.

The preparation process is designed to make the bowel as clear as possible, so a good prep is super important to ensure your gastroenterologist can actually see what's going on in your gorgeous gut. You'll want to know if your gut is showing any inflammation and spot potential changes in the bowel, which might indicate colon cancer. And well, yes, any mention of the big C is scary, but early diagnosis is the key to successful treatment.

### *What to expect*

So let's get super practical. Here are some simple guidelines on what to expect:

- Your medical team will provide you with some dietary guidelines and a drink (usually MoviPrep) to take before your scan. I find the MoviPrep solution is best taken cool, with a little bit of flavoured essence. Having it cool (not cold) makes it a little more bearable, as it disguises the taste. Of course, any added flavouring needs to be transparent so that it doesn't cast any dye into your intestine, which will confuse the clarity of the picture.

- Follow the preparation guidelines carefully so that you don't end up having to repeat the procedure. A low-residue diet (potatoes without skins, well-cooked cauliflower and root veg like carrots) is generally advised in the two days leading up to your scope; high-fibre foods, grains, seeds, nuts and vegetable skins are best avoided as they can hang around in your intestine for a while.

- Once your gut is cleaned out and ready to roll, on the day of your scope, you'll be offered a choice of pain meds. Now, this is personal and best discussed with your consultant or IBD nurse. If you have a severe flare, then you will likely need to be sedated and be out for the count. In one procedure, I got a bit trippy on the meds before they fully kicked in, and I started exclaiming quite loudly how beautiful my colon was. Yep, it was me, and I'd been doing loads of affirmations before the big day. I'm sure my medical team found it entertaining.

- If you are in remission, consider having Entonox (gas and air), then you can take a sneak peek at the display screen. This way, you can get up close and personal with your bowel. Getting familiar with your inner landscape is really handy for gut healing visualizations. You get to see all your hidden world in full technical glory. But if you need to have a sedative, take it. A colonoscopy in flare is a painful experience.

- Base belly breathing (*see page 31*) can help with the level of discomfort. I've been told by doctors – mid-procedure – not to overdo this, as it can make their view of the bowel a little unstable. This shows just how powerful deep base belly breathing can be, creating an inner massage for our gut.

Our gorgeous guts are so often left to pick up the pieces of our lives, so a colonoscopy is a perfect time for some gut-loving affirmations. If you've had a bad experience, it's time for a good gut conversation and a chance to reframe the whole situation. To have the chance to see this precious piece of your internal workings and love it, affirm it – is an honour. Your colonoscopy is a chance to love that colon. And start to care for every inch of that long tender ileum.

There are several different procedures that you may experience in the process of trying to understand what the cause of your gut troubles is. One quite common one is an endoscopy, where a tube with a small camera is inserted down your throat so that your gastroenterologist can check out the upper sections of your digestive tract. Usually, you'll be guided on not eating for several hours pre-procedure. And whilst you may experience a sore throat after the examination, some relaxing deep breathing can help reduce anxiety and discomfort during the procedure. If your doctor opts for a wireless endoscopy, you may get the chance to see the whole of your digestive tract. Whatever your doctor decides, it may be a little while before you get your confirmed diagnosis.

And as an aside, if you've undergone bowel prep for a colonoscopy, it will have a significant impact on your gut microbiome in the short term. Taking this type of preparation can have a pretty dramatic impact on your gut bugs. In one study, 22 per cent of the participants lost the subject-specificity of their microbiota.[10]

So after taking all that gloopy mixture and following a low-residue clear-out before your scope, you'll need to make sure your post-colonoscopy nutrition is supporting you to repopulate your beautiful gut. The good news is that it generally is restored within a couple of weeks post-procedure. Still, it's helpful to be aware of the potential impact and actively support your gut with pre- and probiotics.

So now you've had your colonoscopy, endoscopy or whatever combo of tests your gastro consultant has chosen. Great, well done. I hope it went well and you have a diagnosis that makes sense to you or that you are in remission. If you're in an active flare, no better time for some gut-loving reflection and self-care. Now it's time to connect.

# CHAPTER 15

# YOUR GUT GANG

*'The quality of your attention determines the quality of someone's thinking.'*

NANCY KLINE, AUTHOR AND PIONEER OF THE THINKING ENVIRONMENT

There are so many hard-working doctors and nurses who seek to really listen. Deep, empathetic listening has the power to alter our thinking. Sometimes, when we are unwell or in pain, we are simply too overwhelmed by medical information to take it all in. We need time to process what we need to do. At these times, it's critical to have support and to develop a listening relationship with your medical team and your gastroenterologist.

At this early stage, you can engage your doctor, consultant or nurse in a dialogue by preparing in advance of your appointment.

- Read up and be as informed as you can.
- Prepare some questions. Use the specialist language of your gut if you can from Chapter 1.
- Be powerful in your own gut knowledge. Keep a record of your symptoms and triggers and be ready to share this. (Your journal from Chapters 3 and 10 will help you here.)

- Seek out well-qualified and experienced alternative practitioners, dieticians, nutritionists – folk that you connect with.

## Your wider gut network

Your gut gang is the group you create around you who are your healing allies. They will include your GP, your IBD nurse, your consultant and his/her team.

Having been involved in many coaching conversations, I know how deep listening can help us sustain change. In the spirit of that, I ask you to take a few moments to journal.

### Gut reflecting

Grab your Gut-loving Journal and reflect on the following questions:

- How health articulate do you feel you are on a scale of 1–10?
- What would 10 look like to you?
- Who is in your current gut gang?
- How are you communicating with them?

---

An old patient is better than a new doctor, but only if that patient is invested in their wellness. If you show yourself to be self-aware, with good gut knowledge, gut compassion and commitment to your healing journey, you're in the perfect place to form a partnership with your gut gang. You will be able to approach your medical appointments with greater confidence, curiosity and openness, ready to listen and to co-create the healing journey with your doctor. You are the expert at living in your body, at knowing where the pain is, in what your triggers are. Your knowledge of yourself must not be underestimated in the conversation about your healing journey.

Doctors have years of medical training, enabling them to diagnose and treat the human body, so let their knowledge and wisdom meet with *your lived experience*. In that space, healing can take place. However, in my experience, there are a couple of important areas where the current medical processes fail to meet our gut trouble:

- The deep listening skills to support change and an empowered mindset in the 'patient' – read person.
- The necessary lag time between groundbreaking scientific discoveries and the work it takes to transmute that into approved NICE guidelines and treatment.

Right now, as you read these words, the research on the microbiome is evolving rapidly. How this translates into treatments on the ground takes time. These paradigm shifts that transform the way we see the body and how we treat it evolve over years, even decades. Evidence-based research has clear timelines and constraints. The process has built-in fail-safes. Trials are replicated multiple times before altering the traditional treatment protocol. It takes time.

But in that process, there's a real danger that we lose sight of what we know to be true – that the ways we are living our choices, small and large, each day are part of us getting sick and contribute to our chronic gut troubles. So, yes, whilst fully acknowledging the picture is nuanced and unique to each of us, we have the power – a clear power – to make changes if we have real conversations with the healthcare professionals in our lives. Take a moment to explore how you can develop a partnership with your gut gang and how you can take this partnership a little deeper still in your actual appointment.

## ♥ Gut Love ♥

You may know your GP or consultant really well, or maybe you've just been diagnosed. They may be experts, but so, my dear, are you. Be calm and positive – I know you will.

Take a pad or your journal to your appointments and have your questions ready. Tell them that you want to go through some questions. Here are a few suggestions:

- What do you recommend that I eat for IBD/IBS alongside this medication?
- Can you share what IBD/IBS patients who are thriving with this condition are doing?
- What about the new research on the microbiome? Is it possible my condition is linked to dysbiosis?
- I am seeking to build up my access to pro- and prebiotics to support my microbiome's diversity. What's your view? Have you had other patients where that approach has helped with their symptoms?
- Is stress, anxiety or lifestyle a factor?

## Casting your healing net a little wider

Knowing the language of your body and the specialist language of your illness is a compassionately empowering step. In my gut gang, at various points of my healing journey, I've involved a range of people and practices: nutritionists, dieticians, acupuncturists, healers and more. I know the process of deepening loving-kindness and self-compassion took my healing to a new level. It was this mindset shift that changed everything because, as I've said before:

*Compassion is the bridge between what we know and what we do.*

When selecting an alternative practitioner, I have always gone with my gut. My healing partners tend to be further along the path, and we usually share the same language, but I feel that they have some wisdom to offer. This is why it is important to treat yourself as the expert in your health journey. Research and the best advice are evolving because many factors impact overall health and wellbeing.

It's time to talk, scale out a little wider to think about the other guts in your life.

## Gut network review

Sketch out who is part of your support team. Take out your **Gut-loving Journal**, open it so you have two pages to write across, and place a lovely smiling circle right at the centre of the page – that's you!

1. Now draw little figures or shapes of all those folk who form part of your current gut network. If they are close and supportive, they will be right next to you on here.
2. Who is on the outer fringes of your constellation, who doesn't even know about your gut condition but might be able to offer support?
3. What can you do today to grow your gut network? There are plentiful avenues to connect you with your wider gut gang online. In the Resources (*see page 265*), we'll look at some places for support. There are so many possibilities locally and internationally to connect with gut-loving folk!

## Gut integrity in relationships

Let's talk about the elephant in the room. If you're trying to make some significant changes to your diet and lifestyle, it's going to impact those around you. That's something you're going to need to talk about. Especially if you do the cooking. Because what you really don't want to be doing is creating lots of different dishes. If you're the cook, you want to cook gut-loving recipes for everyone you live with. This may take some deep gut-led conversations.

Food is a big part of family life. In fact, as you embark on a journey to transform your relationship with food, remember food is love and comfort. So you may want to break this particular conversation into several shorter gut-love conversations about your personal food map with your partner, family or housemates. I suggest looking at four key stages:

### *Part 1: The other guts in your life – shopping*

Start with how you shop and how you prepare foods. Explore new places to pick up ingredients. Local, independent health food stores can be a treasure trove of new foods and supplements. Read food labels, and as a plant-based dude, you need to be selective. Get creative with your old favourite recipes, swap out trigger foods and try new ingredients. Get a range of different simple meals you are confident are good for your particular gut.

You'll need to plan ahead for busy times by preparing meals in advance. What's going to be your own gut-loving equivalent of chucking a pizza in the oven. Yeah, it may be a pizza, but it'll be a whole different kind of pizza. Hmm. And by the way you'll almost certainly need to make friends with your freezer.

At this stage in your gut journey, you will be buying and preparing food that nourishes you and heals your gut.

## *Part 2: Your gut-loving food talk – eating out*

Now, this is where it could get complicated. You're in luck. Most places now have a whole section dedicated to gluten-free and dairy-free and all sorts of combos in between. But hold your horses – some of that stuff is no good for your gut.

We know when we are time poor that we tend to be easy, non-selective and superficial. *Well, why the hell not? Everyone is doing it, aren't they?* we say, casting our eyes around the restaurant. But if you've built up a loving relationship with your ileum and colon, you'll be way more motivated to take care of them. If you're out and about, that mindful gut-love is going to cut through, 'I just fancy that hot dog right now.'

Right now, having that hot dog (just like my wife, husband, son, bestie) feels like the most loving thing you can do. You're hungry, and there's a lot of hungry gut bacteria and thousands of years of evolution saying – 'Hell, yes.'

At those moments, and you'll surely have a few, you need to get *really* clear about what that hot dog's journey is going to be in your body. As some IBD folk say: 'A minute on the lips, a lifetime on the toilet.' The atoms in that hot dog, the processed fat molecules, the sticky layers of gluten – they will get right down and dirty with your inflammatory cytokines. And this, my dear, is the kind of stuff you'll need to share with the other guts in your life. You know the guts you live with and those that love you and your gut.

Remember – your intestinal wall is just one cell thick, more delicate than the surface of your eye. How does that hot dog – for hot dog read bagel, biscuit, baguette – look to you right now?

Maybe you feel so strongly that you still want it. Fair enough. You get to choose. And this is the important bit. Tell your gut-loving gang how you want them to support you at that moment. Because it is your decision and as hard as it may be to say no on that occasion, eventually the choice not to eat the stuff you struggle with will be close to effortless. I promise you that. You will be in a place where you have achieved so much clarity, so much gut-loving insight, that you will simply skip past that hot dog like it's poison. You will have a searing sense of clarity and a purpose so strong that the sight of your favourite old foods will not faze you. Sometimes it will be that simple.

However, there may be times when it's harder, and this is where you might want to do a little research. You want to find places that you can visit; venues that are willing to make some simple swaps for you. This is where you become your own gut advocate. So be calm, be confident and be polite – ask everything you need to ask. Share this stuff with your loved ones. If they want to arrange a surprise date night or a big family celebration, you want to make it easy for them to know what's on your food map.

The more you can start to build good gut health conversations with local eateries, the more they can cater to you and your gut, the better. They get a happy, regular customer, and you get to eat out without the sense of restraint you're all too familiar with. Trust that you can find the best version of plenty of tasty meals for you and your gut bugs.

### *Part 3: Your personal food map and family time – celebrations*

First and foremost, food feeds our safety needs. But what we also see is how much food sits at the centre of almost every ritual. From pumpkin pie at Thanksgiving or the symbolic joint cutting of a wedding cake, to the breaking of bread at a Shabbat. Food connects us. Food acts to reinforce our bonds of connection – it links us emotionally and psychologically.

So you're going to want a slice of that birthday cake for sure. And you're going to need to get your head around those situations and have a clear plan. For your own birthday, make the most gorgeous cake you can – swap out and change and tweak that recipe. It's your special day, so think who can help you with this?

## *Part 4: Treats*

This is for you. Your personal food map must include foods you **love**. If you or those around you have the limiting belief that eating healthily is depriving yourself, you will always be fighting your food and yourself.

To integrate gut integrity into our lives, we need to reframe our mindset. So take a breath and start thinking about what you need to share and with whom – your partner, your loved ones and your wider gut gang.

You're here because your gut is troubling you. I know that change happens naturally when you are sick of feeling sick and change stays naturally when you start to feel better. Now you've got strong motivation to change, growing gut-level compassion driving deep integrity – you can do it.

There are many delectable desserts and sugar-free treats that you can buy or make, whatever your personal food map. Experiment, explore and be confident that you can treat yourself and let others do so for you. This psychology will be crucial to sticking with the significant changes you're going to be making. Personally, I couldn't now live without cacao nibs. I chuck them in flapjacks and banana loaf to make whatever I'm baking that extra level of special – because me and my lovely gut are worth it. How about you?

What can you do to bring the sexy stuff back into your personal food choices, a sprinkling of joy in the landscape of change you're making right now?

CHAPTER 16

# THE SUSTAINABLE GUT

*'What will you do with*
*your one wild precious life?'*

MARY OLIVER, PULITZER PRIZE-WINNING POET

If you eat something that doesn't sit well with you – OK, it's done. Graciously and compassionately breathe in and out and take a moment to recommit and reconnect with your gut. We've already explored some of our deepest taboos: good food, bad food – so many labels.

I'm not a fan of the term 'illegal' food, a term used for some restricted diets. Those of us with gut health 'restrictions' need to confidently drop that kind of language and try not to get too hung up about what we can't eat and look at what we can eat. Yes, we're probably giving up many of those dopamine-laden empty junk food calories that have become the 'norm', but that makes it even more important to take a fresh perspective. Now is the perfect time for an expansive exploration of foods from different cultures and cuisines.

## Training your mind and microbes for sustainable change

I've always been fascinated by the disconnect between what we **know** and what we **do**. You know the graveyard of good intentions that never quite made the final cut of our lives? We know compassion is the foundation for gut integrity and acts as a bridge between our knowledge and our actions. However, we also need to pepper this with some mindful self-awareness because our ability to change habits is directly proportional to our increased self-awareness in our own lives.

So, I hope by this stage you've started to spend even a few minutes practising daily mindfulness (*see page 153*). If not, please don't beat yourself up. Just know that studies show that folk like you – who practised mindfulness for as little as eight weeks – had small but noticeable differences in brain activity, levels of calm, and a greater sense of wellbeing.[11] Feeling more motivated?

The fact is, if we don't increase our self-awareness, even when we know better, we can still act out – a little mindlessly – doing stuff that harms us. We may have patterns of self-sabotage or a strong need to rebel or 'treat' ourselves. Sometimes we just act out of habit and familiarity. Then we continue down the old rinse-and-repeat patterns we've always followed.

To make change stick, you need to know your oats from your onions. So time to get out your Gut-loving Journal and write **one** thing. Yes, I'm really specific here, just **one** thing under each of these four headings that you can commit to doing today:

### *1. Start small and keep it simple*

Keep thinking simple, specific and doable. For example, stock your cupboards with foods you love that love you back. Remove foods that trigger your gut. Create a short daily mindfulness and movement practice – a five-minute practice is a good starting point.

### *2. Celebrate your forward motion*

Every time you choose the healthy option over sugar, give yourself a little smile. Each time you complete three deep breaths of mindful awareness, look yourself in the eye and say, 'Great'. We have a tendency to focus on what we've not done rather than celebrate the good stuff. This is about working on our inner self-talk.

### *3. Be compassionately kind to yourself*

Write yourself the most loving affirmation you can think of. Turn your kitchen into the bright, beautiful gut-loving centre of your home. Decorate your bedroom as an oasis of calm. Keep returning to your motivation, to care for yourself and your guts.

### *4. Make it social: Shout out.*

This is where your gut gang and your wider gut network come into play. Share what you are doing – you'll find a wealth of resources, shared recipes and tips from those on the gut health journey.

You've got **four simple things** that are doable today. I'm excited for you to begin. However humble, however insignificant, start today – not tomorrow – but now.

## Compassionate and sustainable change

Go slow and consistent on this path. Most IBD and IBS food protocols suggest building up changes to your diet and lifestyle slowly. You may need to have phased introductions of key food groups, which you try and test. For example, typically, your gut bugs and your sensitive gut may not tolerate high levels of fibre. So you don't want to do things drastically. Even if you are in well-controlled remission. You want to make changes where you can reflect on the impact of lifestyle and food choices. Watch your reactions, keep your food mood tracker up to date (*see page 133*).

Monitor your weight and make sure you are eating sufficiently to keep you strong and healthy. As part of this, keep focused on the energy of your change. How's the relationship with yourself going? How's your inner self-talk? As you move yourself to change, what is the feeling you are sending to yourself and your gut? Be honest, are your off-hand comments casually cruel? How do you speak about your gut? With frustration, irritation? How can you have more authentic discussions about your gut health today?

Time to reflect, take stock and complete a gentle gut check-in.

## The roadmap to gut integrity

As you compassionately commit to removing the old inflammatory triggers, you restore the physical integrity of your gut wall. As you reverse the old vicious cycle of inflammation, low energy and discomfort, you start to feel better. And as you naturally eat a wholesome intuitive diet, you start getting creative about reducing chemicals and pollutants in your environment and spending time outside in places that will nurture your microflora. You move more and create healthy sleep rituals.

As we honour the integrity of our gut instincts, the voice of our intuition grows stronger. We establish emotional gut integrity by tuning to signs of stress and overwhelm early and committing to rituals of self-care. As we grow our gut integrity, we deepen our access to our authentic gut-level emotions through journalling and breathwork.

## The crossroads of gut integrity

Gut knowledge, gut compassion and gut healing are paths that lead us to this crossroads. It is here that we choose our road to an authentic gut-led life. We get to choose.

*Even though the pressures of following food conventions may feel overwhelming, you are being called to follow your gut-led life.*

When our guts are at a crisis point, we may feel drawn to closing down, protecting the tender tissue of our underbelly. We fold, turning inwards to our own pain. In contrast, when our gut is loved and vibrant with health, it feeds our body. We stand tall, whole and energized.

This parallels the healing of the solar plexus chakra (*see page 30*); it feeds our heart's energy and enables us to look beyond ourselves to others. It fuels the energy of self-compassion inwardly and ultimately outwards to others. Gut integrity will ground you in a way that will surprise you over and over.

But let's just remind ourselves we are each unique. My gut integrity may well look different from yours. Mine might be plant-based, gluten-free and grounded in my morning yoga practice. Yours might be about maintaining your J pouch, preventing infections, balancing your energy levels and having a no-sugar diet. Someone else might be about dropping the junk food and creating a more balanced gym routine, with a daily Wim Hof breathing session thrown in for good measure. Hey, we are each unique, carrying our beautifully complex biomes in tow.

Now, as you stand at the crossroads of gut integrity, it's time to start to imagine what this gut-led life will mean. There's a power in imagining the possibilities.

## Roadmap to gut integrity

Let's start with some questions to get you sensory and grounded in the life you seek to create.

- What would physical gut integrity feel like in your body?
- What would emotional gut integrity feel like in your belly?
- What would mental gut integrity sound like when you speak to yourself?
- How would spiritual gut integrity resonate in your body when you wake?
- How can you move towards gut integrity today?

Gut integrity means entering a dialogue with your gut. This inner voice has always been with you. It guided you as a child and shaped some of your big decisions. It's usually in our teens we start to discount it, looking outwards for approval from others.

As you do the work of gut healing and honour the voice of your gut integrity, you will start to feel it nudge you. At first, it may be the merest whisper or a soft flutter in your belly. But it will grow in strength, and as it does, it will align with and nourish both your belly and your heart chakra (*see figure 4, page 30*).

## The journey to deeper gut integrity

Healing is a journey. In Part I you recorded your gut narrative. You captured your past and how you have arrived in our present gut state. You now have the chance to reframe this narrative, to re-envision the next stage of your journey.

In Paulo Coelho's *The Alchemist*, the protagonist must go on a journey towards his dreams. His journey isn't linear but circular. He returns home to discover that his treasure has always been at home, but he could only learn this through his journey.[12]

We are like the hero/heroine in our own journey. Our healing is a journey towards our true self. Towards the wholeness that we long for and lack. We are called to a journey. We may refuse this call out of fear. We can carry on in our own limited life, but once we take a step towards healing, we will be aided in miraculous and often unexpected ways.

There is a kind of inner surrender in illness, a vulnerability (if we are willing to go there). Healing takes place in so many different ways. Even if we choose to release part of our gut through surgery, healing can still occur at an emotional and spiritual level.

*'I'm proud of the scars in my soul. They remind me that I have an intense life.'*

PAULO COELHO, *THE ALCHEMIST*

It's possible to reframe your journey to gut integrity as being a journey towards yourself. Your journey can be as big or small as you want to make it. You have been a warrior, a worrier and a victim. We hold all these different possibilities in ourselves. Sometimes we get stuck in a particular mode of being. Now, as you deepen your gut integrity, you get to write the next part of the journey.

## From gut love letter to gut contract

In Part II you wrote a love letter from your gut and placed it in your Gut-loving Journal (*see page 109*). I want you to revisit your letter now, so you remind yourself of the spirit of the letter and your growing gut love to start to envision the life you want for your gut by creating a mindful vision board.

I have my vision board next to my bed. It's the first thing I glance at in the morning and usually the last thing I see before going to bed. If you've never created one before, it's simple – you just need a few of your favourite magazines, scissors and a glue stick.

There is power in the process. There's a certain energetic intention to the physical process of creating your own board and selecting a place to put it up.

## Gut vision board

There's a certain magic that happens when you start to envision what you long for. Play music, hum affirmations. You'll need a big table or a rug. Surround yourself with inspiration. Trust you are sending out a thread of connection to the things you want to create in your life. By creating a real place for them, you are making space for the possible.

1. Start by placing a picture of yourself glowing with health right at the centre of your board. Be bold and brave with your vision.
2. Ask yourself: What is the life you want for yourself and your gut? Call on your gut love letter (*see page 109*) to inspire you!
3. Imagine a life where you and your gut are in harmony.
4. OK, now create your board with inspirational quotes and words that resonate with you. Every time you see it, breathe and smile, trusting you are moving towards your vision.

## 30-day love your belly challenge

Next, let's explore how to embed change by playing with different ways to show up to the belly in your life in the **30-day love your belly challenge**. There are a few ways to approach this self-compassion challenge. Go for it and commit to spending a month making the whole list. If you are in an active flare, take it slowly and spread the actions by selecting just two or three across a week.

Set yourself up for success, so be ambitious but SMART and realistic. How can you extend this list with your own #Lovethybelly practices so that you build this up towards #loveyourbellyforlife?

## 30 ways to love thy belly

Over the next 30 days, consciously seek to reduce sugar. Avoid eating highly processed foods. Aim to starve out the less helpful bugs in your gut. At the end of the month, you will have started to play with new ways of showing up to yourself, creating hooks for new habits that will love your gut.

1. Let's start with the breath. Commit to breathing deeply today (*see page 31*). Choose cycles of three or seven breaths at key points in your day. Start in the morning first thing. Breathe. Take three breaths before each meal.
2. Morning juicy guts. Start your day with plant power and select one of the juices from Part V (*see page 235*) depending on the season.
3. Feed your microbiome with fibre – chia seeds and psyllium husk are great ways to up your fibre intake (*see page 141*).
4. Splash your face and chest with cold water as soon as you wake up. If you're brave, have a cold shower. This stimulates your vagus nerve, reducing inflammation.
5. Love your prebiotics. Include Jerusalem artichokes, garlic and onions in your food today.
6. Try baby dandelion leaves in your lunchtime salad today. Source and select the youngest leaves.
7. Compassionately caress your jejunum and affirm your ileum.
8. Eat at a table with a tablecloth and cutlery. Have a screen-free meal. Use your senses to enjoy your food, appreciate the smell and textures. Lean in and love your plate.
9. Sort out your sleep hygiene and get an early night (*see page 96*). An overnight fast of at least 14 hours will help your gut rest and recover and nourish those beloved Akkermansia.

10. Send love to your guts by creating your own compassion affirmations (*see page 151*).
11. Bake your own bread – try the bread recipe in Part V (*see page 249*).
12. Carry out a mindful love-thy-belly massage using analgesic oils (peppermint for waking up, lavender and chamomile for sleepy massage, *(see pages 103–104*).
13. Start today with a beautiful yoga sequence (*see page 167*).
14. Chew your food fully until it is the consistency of applesauce. Remember to breathe between mouthfuls. Put your knife and fork down and just focus on your plate.
15. Go cruciferous today – sprouts, broccoli, cabbage.
16. Practice pranayama nose breathing or Wim Hof Method breathing.
17. Complete a Gut Love Dance (*see page 174*). Breathe in your belly and play with all the fluid power of your emotions and energy. Express who you are, who your gut is, and align your body.
18. Aim for 30 different forms of plant-based foods this week* (*see page 225* for inspiration).
19. Breathe in your biome. Take a mindful walk before your lunch today. Even if you only get fresh air for a short time.
20. Spiralize vegetables to replace carbs such as pasta and rice. This will reduce your carbohydrate load and increase your five/eight a day (*see page 226*).
21. Add tasty herbs and spices to your plate today. Try cinnamon on your breakfast oats. It's thermogenic and supports stable blood sugar (*see pages 230–231*).
22. Find time today for stillness – the compassionate practice of non-doing. Spend five minutes without your phone, TV, tablet or laptop.

23. Wake up early, see the sunrise and find a quiet space where you can see a skyline. A hilltop view – this is healing for your mind and gut. Sit and breathe your biome.

24. Make your own fermented foods (*see recipes, page 252*). Try simple sauerkraut or tasty cucumbers.

25. Create rituals around your food (*see page 92*). Say Grace (or your own alternative), sing a little hymn/song of gratitude and bless your food before eating it. Sit after eating and send love to your digestive tract for processing this food

26. Try an organic celery juice this morning. Celery juice is rich in anti-inflammatory luteolin, which is great for your gut.

27. Eat something containing butyric acid – buy high-quality virgin olive oil and dress your salad and veg.

28. Focus on strength training to counteract meds that impact your bones – lunges, squats and star jumps. Remember, exercise supports your inner diversity.

29. Combine pre- and probiotic foods today, e.g. tofu, veg miso soup with a side of brown rice (*see page 141*).

30. Tell your gut just how much you love it. Thank it for all the work it does for you each day.

*If you are in an active flare or already following a specific elimination diet, SCD or anti-inflammatory protocol, adopt these recommendations slowly, so you honour the process and go gently.

As you start this challenge, I send you and your gut so much love. Let the healing begin. If you've reached this point in the book, then you are well on your way to living a compassionate gut-led life.

# GUT INTEGRITY 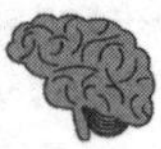

- Celebrate simple changes which you make today and share what you are doing with those who love you and your gut!
- Practise being open with those around you about your gut journey and share some of the changes you are making right now.
- Aim to have a family meal at least once a week which everyone can eat.
- Practise being fully gut articulate by preparing for the next conversation with your medical team and bringing some questions with you.
- Grow your gut gang by connecting to others to support and inspire your journey.

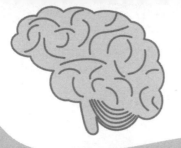

# Part V

# Gut-Loving Food and Recipes

*'Use very simple foods and flavour them fantastically.'*

Chloe Coscarelli, award-winning vegan chef and author

To help you along your way, I'm sharing a few of the plant-based meals that form part of day-to-day life. These are simple, easy-to-make meals, with an emphasis on fresh, seasonal produce and home-grown simplicity.

They are tasty and flexible, so be confident to swap in ingredients that your gut knows you need. Each of our gorgeous guts is unique, so honour yours by mindful eating.

There are no rules here, no forbidden foods, just foods that love and heal your gut and those that don't. And what's super exciting is that 'Food is medicine. We can change our gene expressions with the foods we eat.'[1] Right now is the perfect time to create a personal food map that works for you!

# CHAPTER 17

# FILL YOUR KITCHEN WITH MUSIC AND GUT-LOVING SOUL

*'Let food be thy medicine and medicine thy food.'*

HIPPOCRATES, ANCIENT GREEK PHYSICIAN

Make your kitchen your happy, healthy place. We need to be smart in making gut care as easy as we can, because there's a whole tide of easy, not-so-good gut stuff at the click of an app. And that's what we are competing with. We know there is a fair bit of mindset about how we reframe self-care and 'treating yourself'.

Create a shelf of gut-loving books to choose from. Play music to calm or inspire your creativity. And, well, the kitchen is the perfect place for dancing. In the Ayurvedic system, digestive fire is at its peak around midday. Our cultural patterns tend to move us to eat later in the evening.

Your kitchen is a sensory environment. You have touch, smell, sight, taste and therefore adding the right kind of sound is a key to creating the vibe you want to play in. We've got a pretty small, modern kitchen at home, but we've managed to squeeze in a comfy chair and a couple of stools. It's the perfect place for chatting and catching up at the end of the day. We make sure it's a place that's warm and welcoming.

## Cooking for a calm gut in eight easy steps

Cooking in bulk is great practical gut support. Use the fridge and freezer to stock up and have easy meals ready for days when you simply don't have the time to be in the kitchen for long. Also:

1. Plan ahead by stocking your cupboards, fridge and freezer with gut-loving foods

2. Avoid having foods in your house that aren't gut-loving.

3. Invest in some essential kit, including a blitzer or food processor, pressure/slow cooker, garlic crusher, single side grater/zester, green frying pan, large steel saucepan, glass containers for freezing up batches of food and jars for preserving. If you can, a spiralizer is a fun way of adding extra veg.

4. Aim for a handful of simple meals that you can mix up by adding in different pulses and veg based on seasonality and your very own gut dowsing intuition.

5. Sprout seeds and grow fresh herbs on your kitchen windowsill and use them every day.

6. Learn how to 'treat' yourself and your gut bugs in healthy, happy ways, so you feel food happiness.

7. Learn the simple pleasure of home baking – it is so easy.

8. Experiment with fermenting your own foods.

Follow these guidelines, and you'll effortlessly eat 30 different plant-based foods each week.

## ♥ Practical Stuff ♥

Throughout the recipes, look out for the following symbols:

- Number of plant-based ingredients
- Great for packed lunches or leftovers
- The 3Ps (probiotics, prebiotics and polyphenols)
- ✓ Biome-friendly
- Superfood for an added boost

The recipes are designed to give you some ideas around plant-based, gut-loving diversity. Therefore, they don't strictly follow all the guidelines of either SCD or the IBD-AID. I also use the following abbreviations: GF = gluten-free; DF = dairy-free; YF = yeast-free.

Not all the recipes are suitable if you're in active IBD flare, as it's important to integrate high-fibre ingredients and texture slowly into your healing journey. In fact, if you are in an active flare, I recommend following phase 1 of the IBD-AID diet. Similarly, if you have IBS and haven't yet completed a short eight-week low FODMAP diet, you may wish to complete this first as the recipes are not fully compliant with this food regime.

## Retraining your microbes with mindfulness

In this group of recipes, I want you to see how naturally and easily you can eat at least 30 different plant-based foods each week.

These should include fruit, veg, pulses and nuts. In Jamie Oliver's very readable *Everyday Super Food*, he explores local, seasonal, fresh, diverse cooking in the diets of some of the longest-living humans on the planet. He found plant-based diets are evident in communities around the world with the highest populations of centenarians.[2] The recipes I am sharing are corn-free, dairy-free, gluten-free and yeast-free. These are just to give you a flavour of the simple everyday creativity of foods. They are not all low FODMAP, because whilst going low FODMAP is usually a foundation of IBS healing, it isn't the whole story.

## Grow your own

I'm a passionate advocate for growing your own; it connects us to our food and the cycle of life. If you have kids, it may be a crucial part of their journey to connect them with their plate. Growing is good for our mental health; it is a way to breathe our microbiome and provides easy access to organic foods.

One of the most mindful and grounding things you can do is grow a few pots of herbs. I propagate my basil by buying a good-quality plant and then taking cuttings. Try growing herbs on a windowsill; their green scent will add colour and taste to any dish. Mint, coriander, thyme and basil are all easy on a warmish sill with some sun.

You'll need:

- Good organic (peat-free) compost and a small potting area.
- Seeds – swap seeds at allotments and with friends.
- A sunny ledge, terrace or section of the garden.

If you have more space, and you are up for it:

- Sprout cress, broccoli seeds or chickpeas.

- Grow salads in pots and shallow trays.
- Tomatoes are amazing. They do need TLC and plenty of sun, so grow them on a warm south-facing windowsill.
- Courgettes are so easy to grow in a grow bag in a sunny patch. Like tomatoes, they need watering and care. Courgetti is a fun way of adding veg to your plate.

More space still:

- Potatoes are great if you're short on time and they cope well in large pots. Opt for heritage varieties as they offer greater nutritional benefits.
- Cucumbers just need sunshine and watering but are pretty resilient once the spring frosts are over.
- Apple trees and fruit bushes, like blueberry and raspberry, are low maintenance and great ways of growing your own little packets of organic polyphenol-rich food. Once established, they come back year on year.

## Beautiful Brunches and Breakfasts

These recipes are designed to start your day packed with fibre and to set you on course to eat varied plant-based foods that will love and heal your gut. I aim for diversity, so I am integrating some FODMAPs, but it is also easy to swap out and use alternative ingredients. Fresh herbs pack extra flavour, so use as many as you can in your cooking if you are on an elimination diet.

Breakfast is simply my favourite meal of the day. Brunches generally contain combinations of my most loved ingredients, are a great way to set up your energy, and set your eating course for the rest of the day. Our body needs different fuel types depending on the seasons, so I've shaped the recipes to match the seasons.

## *Summer Bircher Muesli*

Easy breakfast – a deliciously divine way to start the day and takes only minimal prep the night before. IBS- and IBD-friendly.

*Serves 2*
*Prep time: 8 minutes (prepare the night before)*

**Ingredients**

1 cup of oats (GF or steel-cut)
1 generous tbsp of flax seeds/chia seeds
1 large or 2 small apples, grated (peeled if this is a trigger for your IBS or replace with another fruit such as kiwi for the low FODMAP diet)
2 cups DF milk (coconut adds extra sweetness here)
1 tsp Ceylon cinnamon
10 walnuts, chopped
Sprinkle of pumpkin seeds
Handful of fresh blueberries
1 tsp of your favourite nut butter per person, optional

**Directions**

Place the oats, chia/linseeds seeds and apple in the milk. For a zingier taste, replace the apple with either grapefruit or orange juice.

Stir in a tasty teaspoon of cinnamon, cover with a plate and pop in the fridge overnight.

In the morning, stir (you may need to add a splash more milk or a dollop of yoghurt).

Stir in the walnuts and top with pumpkin seeds and blueberries. Add the nut butter (optional) to pack in some extra protein.

8–12 plant-based ingredients

Prep in a travel-friendly glass kiln jar with a lid

Team with a cup of green tea and you've hit your 3Ps

✓ Biome-friendly linseed fibre, walnuts, blueberries

## *Easy Breakfast Porridge*

Need a warming, gorgeously gut-loving start to the day? Oats are soluble-fibre fuel.

*Serves 1*
*Prep time: 8 minutes (prepare the night before)*

**Ingredients**

60g/2oz millet or steel-cut oats
1 tbsp chia seeds
Sprinkle of dried fruit; goji berries and raisins work well (avoid those coated in sulphur dioxide).
200ml/7fl oz filtered water
250ml/8½fl oz DF milk (organic nut milk or coconut work well)
1 plum, halved or a chopped green banana (low FODMAP-friendly)
1 tsp Ceylon cinnamon, optional
1 tbsp psyllium husk for gut motility

**Directions**

Soak the oats, dried fruit and chia seeds in water overnight.

In the morning, stir in your favourite DF milk.

Place the oat mixture in a saucepan on a low heat and cook for 12 minutes until soft and warmed through. Keep stirring to prevent it from sticking to the pan.

Place the plum under a medium grill for around 8–10 minutes or until lightly toasted.

When the oats are cooked, stir in the cinnamon and psyllium husk, and top with the plum or sliced banana.

8 plant-based ingredients

Warming on-the-go fuel for the day. Place in a container if you want to eat breakfast later in the day and ensure your Akkermansia are flourishing from your overnight fast.

✓ Biome-friendly – gut-loving fibre fuel

The humble oat has so much gut-loving fibre goodness!

## *Weekend Brunch*

Who doesn't love a slow belly brunch with a weekend paper? This one is tasty, quick and simple.

*Serves 2*
*Prep time: 15 minutes*

**Ingredients**

200g/7oz scrambled tofu – (eggs if you aren't vegan) I use 100g/3oz per person.
1 tsp vegan butter for creaminess
½ tsp turmeric – a great spice that turns the tofu a lovely yellow colour
¼ tsp black pepper – cooking turmeric with pepper and oil makes the active ingredient curcumin more bioavailable
2 ripe tomatoes, roughly chopped
6 green tops of spring onions, finely chopped
2 cloves garlic, minced (or a drizzle of garlic-infused oil if you are following the low FODMAP diet)
Handful of fresh coriander or parsley, chopped

**To serve**

1–2 thick slices of soda bread or sourdough bread, toasted

1 small avocado per person, peeled and destoned, and mashed with lime juice (or swap out for lightly steamed spinach/kale)
Side for extra gut love – 1 tbsp plus of your favourite fermented pickle
Drizzle of extra virgin olive oil – go for cold-pressed and quality
Sprinkle of sprouted broccoli seeds

**Directions**

Mash the tofu and vegan butter with the turmeric and black pepper in a pan over a low heat for 3 minutes or until the tofu starts to brown lightly.

Add the chopped tomatoes and the lighter green chopped stalks of the spring onions to the pan and stir. Keep an eye on the pan for a further 3 minutes.

Add the crushed garlic to the pan and cook through for a further 2 minutes. Finally, turn off the heat and add the coriander and remaining darkest green spring onions and stir through.

Top the toasted soda bread with the avocado and a few sprigs of chopped coriander.

To dress the plate, drizzle with a glug of olive oil and a sprinkle of broccoli seeds. Add a dollop of fermented pickle, and you're ready to go.

12–15 plant-based ingredients

All your 3Ps by mid-morning!

✓ Biome-friendly gut-loving diversity

Avocado contains omega and good fats

## *Pancake Heaven – GF DF*

Saturday morning is pancake day in our house. They are joyously simple and can be seasonably updated with your choice of gut-friendly fruit. I tend to have a supply of applesauce to hand as we have a little Pink Lady tree in our back garden. You can use chia/flax seeds to create a chia egg to help bind the ingredients, but honestly, a banana will do the trick. In winter, I tend to add some dried fruit to the mix – cranberries are our favourite. For a festive twist, grate a little dark chocolate over a few orange segments. Yes, a pancake really can suit any season!

*Serves: 3–4*
*Prep time: 20 minutes*

**Ingredients**

100g/3oz flour mix: oat/almond – amazing grains in combo (or buckwheat if you can tolerate it)
1 large green banana
300ml/10fl oz coconut milk for natural sweetness
½ tsp of organic coconut oil
1 tbsp of chia seeds

**To serve**

A portion size of chunks of pineapple (80g/2¾oz), blueberries (80g/2¾oz) and raspberries (80g/2¾oz)
1 lemon, juice and zest (organic lemons are unwaxed – the best choice for zesting)
Sprinkle of your favourite nuts and seeds (walnuts and pumpkin seeds for me!)
1 dollop of kefir-based yoghurt or coconut yoghurt per person
2 tbsp tahini

**Directions**

Blitz the flour, banana and DF milk before stirring in the chia seeds. Leave the mixture to stand for 5 minutes to let the chia seeds soften and expand. The mixture should have a batter-like consistency; add in a little more liquid or flour if needed.

Warm a smidgen of coconut oil in a green frying pan. Cook the pancakes one by one by placing a large tablespoon of pancake mix in the pan at a time (aiming for a disc around 10cm/4in across). Cook each pancake for a few minutes on each side or until golden brown. Pile on a warm plate while you finish cooking the rest of the pancakes.

Sprinkle each pancake with pumpkin seeds for an omega boost and pack your plate high with your favourite fruit. Serve with yoghurt, nut butter or tahini for extra protein.

10 plant-based ingredients

3Ps perfection!

✓ Biome-friendly fibre boost

Berries are super anti-inflammatory gut goodness!

## Seasonal Smoothies

To meet your 30 different plants each week, it's all about smoothie love. If you haven't got the kit to do this, invest in a blitzer. It's a surprisingly easy way to bring more fruit and veg into your day. Our gut bugs love fibre. Using a blitzer rather than a juicer, you are getting the whole benefit of the plant fibre. Seeds are generally fine too. So – bonus – limited chopping and prep.

I tend to use filtered water (to reduce chemical residue) or plant milk. Ensure when adding linseed or psyllium husk that you drink plenty of fluid (water or tea) in an hour or two afterwards. I'm also keeping these simple – you can add and experiment, but in the morning, sometimes simple is best. Bonus – you can leave your house already having had four or five of your five a day (remember five a day is a minimum aim). Each recipe is designed for two healthy smoothies; just place all the ingredients in your blender and blitz to your preferred consistency.

### *Spring Simple Super Green*

18g/¾oz linseed – omega-rich bulking
100g/3oz celery –source organic if possible. Alternatively you can use 100g/3oz kale if you're following the low FODMAP diet.

1 kiwi (I keep the skin on but tend to chop off the hard nub ends)
1 tsp spirulina – use sparingly, as it has a strong taste and will turn this smoothie a brilliant forest green
Filtered water or fresh coconut water for a little extra flavour

4 plant-based ingredients

✓ Biome-friendly

## *Summer Smoothie*

100g/3oz fresh or frozen blueberries.
1 apple – home-grown if you can (you can swap this for 1 peeled papaya if you're following the low FODMAP diet)
Large handful of spinach – organic
1 tbsp rosehip – UVA protective
5g/⅛oz prebiotic fibre mix (Chuckling Goats' Complete Prebiotic is my favourite go-to; it works well with berries as it has a natural grey tone)

4+ plant-based ingredients

✓ Biome-friendly

## *Autumn Aches*

1 carrot
1 apple, skin on (you can swap this for 1 peeled orange if you're following the low FODMAP diet)
1 tbsp maca powder
5–6 walnuts
Handful of fresh mint leaves

5 plant-based ingredients

✓ Biome-friendly

### *Winter Fill Me Up*

1 green banana
5–6 dates/figs for natural sweetness (or swap for 6 frozen strawberries if you're following the low FODMAP diet)
12 almonds
200ml/7fl oz warmed almond milk, infused with either a small nub of ginger or 1 crushed cardamom pod
2ml/0.07 fl oz ginseng
1 tsp chia seeds

5 plant-based ingredients

✓ Biome-friendly

## Gut-soothing soups

Soup is one of the simplest ways of packing plant-based foods into your week. Add a slice of warm homemade bread, and you've got a match made in heaven.

In summer, I love a zingy green pea soup; for autumn and winter, the warmer, heavier flavours of squash and root vegetables. The trick is to have a good-sized cast iron pan or invest in a pressure cooker and make plenty. Soup making is a serious business, and you'll be able to batch cook and create delicious lunches with ease.

### *Fresh Summer Soup*

This is a divinely delicate summer soup. To retain the bright green colour and vitamin C, cook with a light touch. Alongside the gut-loving fibre, peas provide a handy source of plant-based iron. It's best served straight away.

*Serves 4*
*Prep time: 20 minutes*

**Ingredients**

450g/1lb frozen or fresh peas (or swap for 450g/1lb green beans)
Generous handful of fresh mint (take the leaves off the woody stems)
1L/1¾ pints filtered water
1 tbsp fresh miso stock
1 large avocado, peeled and destoned (optional; to make it extra creamy)

**To serve**

1 slice of soda bread per person (*see recipe on page 249*)
A generous dollop of DF yoghurt or kefir per soup portion
100g/3oz mix pumpkin and sunflower seeds
100g/3oz chickpeas, drained
Grind of black pepper

**Directions**

Add the seeds to a warm flat pan and gently toast for around 2 minutes, then place them on a plate ready for dressing. Now drain the chickpeas, season with black pepper and place them in a warm flat pan to toast slightly. Keep an eye on them whilst you start the soup.

Add the peas and water to a pan and bring to a boil. Leave to simmer for 4–5 minutes until the peas are tender and still bright green.

Reduce the heat and add the mint. Stir this through, then add the avocado.

Take off the heat and add the miso paste.

Blitz into a smooth greeny velvety loveliness.

Top with a sprinkle of toasted chickpeas and seeds.

7–8 plant-based ingredients

Make extra and take to work

Miso is a lovely source of phytoestrogens and fermented food. Add in towards the end of the cooking so as not to kill off the good bugs.

✓ Biome-friendly

Peas hold a superfood status for their antioxidant and anti-inflammatory properties!

## *Warming Root Veg Soup*

Soups are a great way of mixing up your pulses. Most pulses need a little more prep time and a soak the night before or a good pressure-cook, so some planning is required. Given it takes time, the best approach is to cook larger quantities than you need, freeze some and use extra for the next day's lunch. Add a splodge of DF yoghurt or kefir for an extra creamy texture. The gut-loving formula: **Soup = pulse + veg + flavour = simple**.

*Serves 4*
*Prep time: 55 minutes*

**Ingredients**

400g/14oz Adzuki or kidney beans canned (or, better, 120g/4¼oz dried Adzuki beans or kidney beans, drained, rinsed and cooked to packet instructions. If following the AID diet, you may need to go slow with pulses. If following the low FODMAP diet, you can use black beans instead.)
3 sweet potatoes, scrubbed and roughly chopped (or if you are going home-grown, easy growers are pumpkin or butternut squash)
1 large red pepper, halved and deseeded
1 tsp smoked paprika
½ tsp turmeric
½ tsp ground black pepper
300ml/10fl oz vegetable stock
Sprinkle of Kombu seaweed (optional – stirred in at the end for an umami base note)
4 green tops of spring onions, chopped to dress
Generous grated nub of ginger
Sprinkle of sprouted broccoli seeds

**Directions**

If using dried pulses, start by cooking them according to the packet directions and set them aside.

Roast the sweet potatoes in a preheated oven (180°C/356°F/gas mark 4) for 40 minutes or until they have softened, started to brown and gone a little crinkled at the edges. Add the red pepper to the oven for the last 20 minutes.

Allow your cooked pulses, roasted sweet potatoes and red pepper to cool a little before blitzing together with the paprika, turmeric and black pepper.

Add the blitzed goodness to a large pan with the vegetable stock and bring to a slow simmer.

Add the lighter green spring onion stems to the simmering soup and reserve the darker green leafy bits for dressing and added crunch. Give the stems five minutes to soften up.

Throw in the grated ginger; feel free to add more to your taste. Simmer gently for a further 5 minutes to let these flavours blend before adding the Kombu seaweed.

Ladle into bowls, then top with the chopped spring onions and sprouted broccoli seeds.

6–7 plant-based ingredients

Keep hot in a flask to enjoy at work for that soothing taste of home

Try Kombu fermented foods

✓ Biome-friendly

Turmeric is a golden base-noted spice that has proven anti-inflammatory qualities

## *Gut-loving Simple Salad Dressing*

Be playful – swap around and play with ingredients based on your new gut dowsing instincts and seasonality. This dressing adds a zingy fermented tang to any salad.

*Serves: 2 for main or 4 for side*
*Prep time: 5 minutes*

### Ingredients

2 tbsp/1fl oz apple cider vinegar – fermented goodness
3 tbsp/1½fl oz cold-pressed olive oil – this is one ingredient where you need to buy the best
1 large clove of crushed garlic (skip the apple and garlic if you are on the low FODMAP diet)
Generous grind of pepper
1 grated apple
Squeeze of lemon for extra zing

### Directions

Place all the ingredients in a glass bottle with a tight lid.

Shake vigorously until the dressing forms an opaque liquid.

5 plant-based ingredients

Go for organic; unfiltered raw ACV is a gut-loving superfood!

✓ Biome-friendly

## *Warming Autumnal Salad*

Salads are super summer fuel; but when the weather turns a little cooler it's time to warm up your salad palette with a little more weight, high protein quinoa and seasonal butternut squash to ground your gut.

*Serves 2 for main or 4 for side*
*Prep time: 1 hour 15 minutes*

**Ingredients**

- 100g/3oz quinoa, cooked
- 1 lemon, zest and juice
- 1 large butternut squash, cut into rough chunks. If you're following the low FODMAP diet, swap for 1 large sweet potato.
- Drizzle of olive oil
- 120g/4¼oz sprouts, thinly sliced – go cruciferous, leave these raw or if that's not quite to your taste sauté in a hot, dry pan for 2 minutes to soften
- 100g/3oz mixed dandelion and rocket leaves
- 1 small courgette, spiralized – fit the straight blade to create ribbons of thin courgette or swap out for cucumber for a fresher taste
- 80g/2¾oz lightly toasted nuts – mix this up – walnuts and sunflower seeds work well

**Directions**

Cook the quinoa to the packet instructions. For zing, add the whole zest and juice of one lemon as it cools.

Drizzle the cubed butternut squash with olive oil and place in a preheated oven (200°C/392°F/gas mark 6) for 35 minutes.

Once cooked, combine the quinoa with the roasted butternut squash, sprouts, salad leaves and courgette.

Sprinkle with toasted nuts.

10 plant-based ingredients

✓ Biome-friendly

Go cruciferous: high in phytonutrients, these superfoods pack a punch of gut-healthy goodness.

## Mindful Mains

These mindful mains are simple, filling and tasty. The recipes are designed to pack a gut-loving punch of your 30 different plant-based foods each week. Remember, diversity is your gut's friend, and fibre, your dear microbes' ally.

### *Lentil Dhal*

This simple staple of Indian cooking is a delicious way of packing more pulses and veg into your diet. I like a mild dhal with warming back notes of heat, but you can add more spice if you prefer.

*Serves 4*
*Prep time: 40 minutes*

**Ingredients**

1 tsp coconut oil or olive oil
1 large red onion, chopped finely
Large nub of ginger, grated
½ tsp cumin
1 tsp garam masala
½ tsp turmeric
½ tsp mustard seeds
½ tsp ground black pepper
1 tsp coriander seeds, crushed
4 cardamom pods, crushed
½ large chilli, deseeded and chopped– keep the white stuff (highest levels of antioxidants)
200g/7oz dry lentils, rinsed
400g/14oz organic plum tomatoes, tinned
400g/14oz coconut milk for an extra creamy note, optional
500ml/18fl oz filtered boiled water
200g/7oz green chopped veg of your choice: spinach or Swiss chard
Stir in the juice of fresh lemon at the end to lift and enhance the flavours

**To serve**

200g/7oz brown rice (high-fibre nutty taste), cooked to packet instructions

Generous handful of fresh coriander to dress

2–3 tbsp cucumber raita (mix together 200ml/7fl oz DF yoghurt (coconut or plain) with 15cm/6in cucumber, finely chopped

Sprinkle of fennel seeds

1 tbsp (homemade) pickled papaya chutney, optional – for fermented goodness

**Directions**

Cook the brown rice to the packet instructions, usually around 25 minutes.

While the rice is cooking, add the onion and the smallest amount of oil to a large pan over medium heat.

Once the onion is softened, add your spices. As they start to release their flavours, stir with a wooden spoon and add the lentils and hot water with the tomatoes.

Once the mixture has come to a slow simmer, reduce the heat and cover for 18 minutes, stirring occasionally.

Stir in the coconut milk (optional) and simmer for a further 5 minutes.

Add the spinach and cover the pan for 2–3 minutes until the leaves are soft and wilted.

Serve the dhal on top of the rice, and sprinkle with fennel seeds. Serve with cucumber raita and a spoonful of chutney.

15 plant-based ingredients

Make extra and take to work

Boost the gut-loving Ps with fermented mango chutney

Green leafy vegetables are firmly in the superfood category. Kale and chard have more texture than spinach, so you might want to cut out the harder stems; all pack a superfood punch of phytonutrients.

*Tip:* Red onions have higher levels of polyphenols than white or brown varieties.

*Fibre extras:* Swap out brown rice for quinoa to mix up your grains.

## *Vegan Bolognese*

This vegan take on an Italian classic is a tasty, easy one-pot meal that you can serve with your choice of pasta or spiralized vegetables. This is a recipe I cook in bulk. Pop in a glass container in the fridge and, after marinating for 24 hours, it's even tastier. To make the most of the flavours of this recipe, serve with a simple side salad of rocket leaves dressed with my Gut-loving Simple Salad Dressing (*see recipe on page 241*) and topped with toasted sunflower and pumpkin seeds. Finish with a sprinkle of sprouted broccoli seeds (these are a true superfood, helping the body to create sulforaphane, which has anti-inflammatory and anti-cancer properties).

*Serves 4*
*Prep time: 40 minutes*

**Ingredients**

1 large red onion, finely diced
300g/10½oz mushrooms, finely chopped – these form the heart of this dish; mix up your buttons with cremini, portobello or porcini. If you're following the low FODMAP diet, you can use oyster mushrooms.
1 large or 2 small carrots, finely diced
2 sticks celery, finely diced
4 large cloves of garlic, crushed – use the crush-and-wait method to enhance the sulphide compounds; 10–15 minutes is ideal. You can swap for a drizzle of garlic-infused oil for the low FODMAP diet.
400g/14oz whole plum tomatoes, tinned – try and go organic if you can (plus half a can of water)
1 large red and 1 large yellow pepper, roasted and diced
1 generous tsp of capers, finely crushed
2 tbsp tomato puree
Generous glug of balsamic vinegar

60g/2oz GF pasta, cooked to packet instruction – vary your grains, as most GF pasta is corn or rice-based. Try whole buckwheat, lentil or chickpea to mix up your plant-based goodies.
Generous bunch of thyme – fresh leaves stripped from woody stems
Generous handful of basil
Grate of parmesan cheese or vegetarian/vegan alternative
Drizzle of cold-pressed organic olive oil

**Directions**

Lightly sauté the onion in a small amount of olive oil. Add the mushrooms.

Once the mushrooms start to brown, add the carrots, leeks and peppers and stir in the tomatoes and puree, plus a splash of red wine if you wish.

Simmer gently on the hob for 10 minutes, then add the garlic and balsamic vinegar. Continue to simmer until the vegetables are tender.

In the meantime, cook the pasta to the packet directions. Once the pasta is cooked, drain but reserve a couple of tablespoons of the cooking water. Combine the pasta and the sauce, and then add the reserved cooking water to loosen the sauce if required before stirring in the thyme.

Sprinkle the fresh basil leaves and cheese over the top of the pasta dish. Drizzle with the best olive oil you have.

12–15 plant-based ingredients

Make extra and take to work. Chilling and reheating pasta reduces its glycaemic index by turning carbs into prebiotic-resistant starch, which our bodies treat as fibre.

A splash of apple cider vinegar at the end and you've got your 3Ps tastily packaged in one dish!

✓ Biome-friendly

Cold-pressed organic olive oil has a rich green colour and a vibrant, almost spicy flavour. It is filled with so much gut-loving, anti-inflammatory goodness. Invest in an expensive high-quality oil in the name of gut love.

*Tip:* Mushrooms are an amazing source of vitamin D, and simply leaving them on a sunny windowsill can boost this essential nutrient.[3] The best mushrooms for high nutrients are portobello or chestnut, which have twice as much immune-boosting chitin as button mushrooms.

## *Spring/Summer Falafel with Guacamole and Lentil Flatbreads*

This is the perfect picnic buffet-style meal. We eat with our eyes first, helping us to get our salivary glands flowing. There is something about having a small plate and topping it up with different dishes that really gets you in the mindful food flow. This is a dish just asking you to dress your table or picnic blanket with beautiful bowls and dishes.

*Serves 3–4*
*Prep time: 25 minutes (the lentil flatbreads need to be prepped 8 hours in advance)*

**Ingredients**

- 800g/1lb 12oz chickpeas, canned, drained and rinsed (or pressure-cook your own)
- 80g/2¾oz mixed nuts (almonds, walnuts, etc.)
- 1 tsp cumin
- Generous handful of parsley
- 4 green tops of spring onions, finely chopped
- Generous handful of fresh mint (leaves removed from the woodiest part of stems), blitzed
- 100g/3oz almond (AID) or buckwheat flour
- 30ml/1fl oz olive oil
- 90ml/3¼fl oz of filtered water, enough to just combine the roughly blitzed ingredients

**For the guacamole**

- 2 ripe avocados, mashed
- Generous handful of chopped coriander with stems and leaves

1 large ripe tomato, chopped into chunks
Sprinkle of chilli flakes (optional, for heat)
1 large lime, juiced.

**Flatbreads**

100g/3oz lentils, soaked in 200ml/7fl oz filtered water for 4–8 hours, drained and rinsed.
100ml/3½fl oz of water
1tsp turmeric
1 tsp paprika
¼ tsp black pepper

**To serve**

2–3 tbsp DF tzatziki (make your own with 200ml/7fl oz creamy DF live yoghurt combined with 20cm/7.8in of finely chopped cucumber, 1 large minced garlic clove, the juice of half a lemon, and a sprinkle of salt for seasoning.)
1 tbsp fermented cucumber (*see recipe on page 253*)
200g/7oz quinoa cooked in 400ml/14fl oz coconut milk
2 tbsp pistachios, crushed for extra wow (you can use pumpkin seeds instead if following the low FODMAP diet)
1 tsp pomegranate seeds

**Directions**

Place all the falafel ingredients in a food mixer and pulse until the mixture starts to clump (don't overdo, or it will be tough).

Mould into small golf ball-sized patties between lightly oiled hands and shape between your palms. If the mixture is too wet, add a little extra buckwheat. If too dry, add a little more water.

Place on a baking tray and put in a preheated oven (190°C/374°F/gas mark 5) and bake for 20 minutes or until golden brown. Turn off the oven when the falafel is cooked, cover and then return to the just warm oven.

Meanwhile, place the quinoa in a pan with the coconut milk and cover. Bring to a light boil, reduce the heat and simmer for a further 20 minutes.

To make the lentil flatbreads, add all the ingredients to a blender and blitz to make a gloopy batter. In a green pan, add a little oil and pour in a ladle of the flatbread mixture. Keep the flatbreads thin and flip over as soon as they are cooked through. Again, these can be left in a warm oven on greaseproof paper whilst you complete the next steps.

To make the guacamole, place your avocado in a wide bowl and stir in the tomato, coriander and lime.

Sprinkle over the pistachios and pomegranate seeds and serve with tzatziki and fermented cucumber.

- 10–12 plant-based ingredients
- Add a dollop of live homemade tzatziki and you're packing in all 3Ps into this tasty little number!
- ✓ Biome-friendly
- Quinoa contains all nine essential amino acids; it's one of the most nutritious foods you can eat and it's high in fibre.

## *Simple Homemade Bread*

I love bread. I've experimented with many GF options over the years, and I am a firm believer in 'bake your own'. I tend to bake on a Sunday morning and then slice and freeze half the loaf for the rest of the week. It's a mindful activity that fits well with the rhythm of Sundays. It has the bonus of the house smelling of beautiful fresh bread to start the week. I recommend using a good-quality GF brown bread flour (Doves Farm is my go-to for high-quality, organic, local product). This bread is wheat-free, gluten-free, and yeast-free.

*Serves: 1 loaf*
*Prep time: 45 minutes*

**Ingredients**

450g/1lb mixed GF brown flour (for the AID diet, go for 300g/10½oz of oat flour and 150g/5½oz almond flour)

50g/1¾oz oats – if you are tolerant, heritage grains like einkorn/spelt or buckwheat are great to experiment with

1 tsp baking soda

400ml/14fl oz DF buttermilk made from 400ml/14fl oz organic soya milk (or a creamy DF milk) with 1 lemon, juiced – option for veggies to add 40ml/1½fl oz of kefir (I recommend ethically sourced from Chuckling Goat) to the mix, as this adds a lightness and a distinctive taste.

**Directions**

Heat the oven to 200°C/392°F/gas mark 6 and pop in a baking tray lined with parchment paper to warm.

Place dry ingredients in a mixing bowl and add in the homemade buttermilk. Combine together gently and firmly – this is a no-knead bread. The mixture will be quite wet and sticky – that's fine.

Shape the bread straight onto your warm baking tray. Shape into a circle with your hands, then use the back of a knife to make a cross on the top.

Bake in the oven for 40 minutes. Allow the bread to cool and then slice.

4 plant-based ingredients

Great sliced for a healthy lunch or with a bowl of soup

✓ Biome-friendly; GF, DF, YF

*Tip:* This bread goes great with a dip. I love hummus – it's a great all-year-round dip that can be mixed up and varied. Chickpeas are naturally super creamy. I like to add in lemon and zest, a generous glug of olive oil, coriander too. For a super-decadent dressing, top with pomegranate seeds, roasted red peppers and shredded herbs.

## *Homemade Oatcakes*

These delicious oatcakes are great as an accompaniment to a bowl of soup or spread with hummus.

*Serves: 12 oatcakes*
*Prep time: 45 minutes*

### Ingredients

220g/7¾oz oats, blitzed into a fine powder
65g/2¼oz melted vegan butter
95ml/3½fl oz filtered water
½ tsp bicarbonate of soda
½ tsp salt
10g/¼oz chia seeds (soak for 3 mins before adding)

### Directions

Preheat the oven to 150°C/302°F/gas mark 3.

Combine all the ingredients in a bowl to form a stiff dough.

Divide the mixture in half and then half again and create 12 small balls.

Press each ball flat with the back of a spoon onto your baking sheet and place in a preheated oven for 30 minutes. Best served warm straight from the oven.

2 plant-based ingredients

These are a super portable little number, topped with some nut butter for a mid-morning snack!

✓ Biome-friendly GF, DF, YF

# *Easy Sauerkraut*

If you have never fermented, start with a cabbage – green or white, you choose. Or maybe a little combo. I like to do a batch of fermenting in one go to use up the brine solution, and have my jars ready. You can use recycled jars for this, but the best ones are glass with easy-release lids. Just make sure you have cleaned them thoroughly and rinse them in boiling water. You'll also need a clean boiled pebble that fits in the top of the jar to weigh down your cabbage.

*Prep time: 20 minutes plus 10–15 days fermenting time*

**Ingredients**

1L/1¾ pints 2 per cent brine solution: 1L/1¾ pints of filtered water + 20g/¾oz sea salt

1 small whole organic red cabbage, finely shredded – grow your own if you can

5g/⅛oz sea salt to rub into the cabbage

5cm/2in finger of ginger, peeled and finely chopped

1 tbsp caraway seeds

1 tbsp of ground peppercorns

**Directions**

Prepare your jar for fermenting. Make sure your hands and everything that comes into contact with the cabbage are clean. Remove any outer damaged cabbage leaves and the tough inner stems. Shred finely and keep a large leaf back ready for the end.

Place the cabbage in a large bowl and spend 5 minutes massaging the salt into the cabbage and ginger. Take a break – you'll start to notice the cabbage liquid in the base of your bowl – then return and continue for another 5 minutes.

Pack the cabbage into the large, sterilized jar with a clean wooden spoon, and sprinkle a few of the caraway seeds and peppercorns as you go.

Cover the mixture with the leaf you kept back at the start.

Top this up with your brine mix.

Now place a pebble on top to hold the cabbage under the liquid. This is where you really need a glass jar (if you use a metal lid, be extra careful that the liquid doesn't touch this, as it will cause a reaction).

Now for the magic wait. After 24 hours, you'll spot a few bubbles rising. Check the cabbage is still under the liquid. Close it up again and keep an eye on it. Is it all submerged? Yes. Any air needing to be released? After around 10 days, it's time to taste it. Ensure the temperature cools to around 18–20°C (64°F–68°F), and the room is dark. For a sourer, more fermented taste, wait 2–6 weeks.

Once you open and start to use it, store in the fridge for up to 6 months – this will slow down any further fermentation and stop any unwanted bacteria from growing. As long as your cabbage isn't mouldy or discoloured, it's fine to eat.

5 plant-based ingredients

✓ Biome-friendly

## *Fermented Cucumber*

When you grow your own cucumber, you will know the sweet secret to happy salads. This is super easy, and it is great as a side for the mains I have included here. It is a super refreshing ferment as a side with curry or falafel.

Ideally, use a pretty glass jar for this with a flip-top lid.

*Prep time: 5 minutes plus 5 days fermenting time*

**Ingredients**

1 small homegrown organic cucumber or half a shop-bought cucumber. You want enough to pack your jar tightly.

Sprig of dill

1L/1¾ pints 2 per cent brine solution (this is 1L/1¾ pints of filtered water + 20g/¾oz sea salt

**Directions**

Halve the cucumbers, keep the skin on and pack in your jar.

Add the sprigs of fresh dill and pour over the brine solution. Weigh down well with a pebble.

When you put the lid on, you will need to either leave it a little loose or remember to check and release pressure as the $CO^2$ will develop and small bubbles will form.

Leave the jar in a dark cupboard to ferment. Keep an eye on it. It will be delicious after around four to five days.

2 plant-based ingredients

✓ Biome-friendly

## Desserts and Treats

A few tasty, quick treats are always handy to have around – just what you need when you are tempted by more processed sugary snacks.

### *Tasty Treat Flapjacks*

Flapjacks can be oh so simple or super special. For extra indulgence, add dark chocolate chunks.

*Serves: 9 generous slabs*
*Prep time: 40 minutes*

**Ingredients**

80g/2¾oz dates, crushed and melted in 80ml/3fl oz coconut oil

4 tbsp/2¼fl oz maple syrup or raw honey
200g/7oz ground oats, blitzed for 3 seconds to make a little powdery oat flour
2 tbsp ground linseed
2 tbsp chia seeds; soak these in a little water or a small mashed banana before you add them – as they absorb a lot of moisture and can make your flapjacks brittle
2tbsp pumpkin seeds
1 tbsp flaked almonds
20g/¾oz cacao nibs (you can add extra if like me, you love these)
20g/¾oz dried fruit – cranberries or goji berries

**Directions**

Preheat the oven to 200°C/392°F/gas mark 6 and line a shallow baking tray with baking parchment. I tend to dot a few spots of melted coconut butter to ensure the parchment sticks.

Mix the maple syrup, dates and coconut oil in a pan over a low heat until warmed and melted.

Combine the rest of the dry ingredients (except the cranberries, cacao and almonds) in a bowl and then add the maple syrup mixture and mix to an even consistency. Once well combined, stir through the cranberries, cacao and flaked almonds until distributed evenly.

Press the mixture into the base of the tray and bake for 22 minutes.

Cut into nine even slabs while still warm.

9 plant-based ingredients

Store in an airtight container for up to four days.

Goji berries are a super-duper food, sometimes called red diamonds; they contain 18 different amino acids.

*Tip:* If you feel like an extra indulgent treat, replace the cacao nibs with dark chocolate pieces (85 per cent cocoa).

# *Banana, cacao and vanilla ice cream*

The secret to healthy summer desserts is all about frozen bananas.

*Prep time: 10 minutes plus 6 hours freezing time*

**Ingredients**

3 large bananas – mix green (extra fibre and low FODMAP) and ripe ones
100g/3oz of soaked cashews (leave to soak in filtered water for four hours, then drain). You can swap in macadamia nuts if following a low FODMAP diet.
2 tbsp of cacao powder
½ tsp vanilla bean extract

**To serve**

12 pecans, lightly toasted and chopped
Raspberry, chia and date compote (100g/3oz raspberries, 2 tbsp chia seeds, and 60g/2oz dates mashed together and warmed through in a pan)

**Directions**

Blitz the bananas until smooth – or mash well with a fork. Add in your drained cashews. Stir in the cacao powder and mix thoroughly, then add a splash of vanilla extract.

Place in an airtight freezer container for at least six hours or overnight. Scoop into bowls and serve with raspberry, chia and date compote.

For a more vanilla taste, leave out the cacao and keep it simple, or add chopped nuts – I personally love pecans. Stir in some cinnamon for creamy yellow ice cream and drizzle with raspberry chia compote.

8 plant-based ingredients

✓ Biome-friendly

- Chia seeds make a high-protein, high-calcium and iron-rich food source

### ♥ Gut Love ♥

Looking for some gut-loving inspiration? Get to know your carminative herbs. Have in a cuppa or add to your food. Carminatives are ancient traditional remedies. The oils in these herbs stimulate the digestive system and support good gut health. Their main action is to soothe and settle the gut wall. They have been used traditionally to ease gas from the digestive tract. Great to have as a post-meal cuppa.

## Simple anytime and post-meal warmers

Hot milk in the evening is a great go-to. Turmeric latte has a warming base note, so it's not for everyone. If you fancy trying it, add a small teaspoon to a cup of plant-based DF nut milk heated on the stove and sweeten it with maple syrup, a grind of black pepper and even a dash of vanilla extract. Another favourite of mine is hot cacao nib chocolate with warming nutmeg milk. It's as simple as melting the nibs in the milk of choice with grated nutmeg to taste.

**Nutmeg** is a mood-boosting and digestive aid, perfect for cold evenings. Other spices to try:

**Cloves** are the stars of polyphenols. Packed with antioxidants, anti-inflammatory, antiseptic and anti-flatulence – handy if you trip up and eat a trigger food. Particularly good with baked apples.

**Coriander** – love or loathe – is packed full of antioxidants.

**Fennel seeds** are frequently eaten in Indian cuisine after a meal to aid digestion.

**Ginger** is a digestion-boosting herb. This warming spice is great for heating up the digestive system and adding seasonal warmth to protect against autumn and winter colds. Ginger's anti-inflammatory compounds rescue joints and muscle ache, which is common for those of us with IBD.

**Turmeric** is an on-trend spice because it's a proven powerhouse of anti-inflammatory support, great for digestion and immune functioning. Pack in as much as you can tolerate. To be bioavailable, the spice requires warming and heating through cooking, so great to add to curry.

# A GORGEOUS AUTHENTIC GUT FOR LIFE

Waking up to your life and your gut is a journey. A journey that you may have to recommit to over and over again. I hope that the exercises and practices shared have deepened your gut wisdom and intuition – return to them as often as you wish. Keep growing those gut instincts.

If right now your gut is struggling, commit to giving it the care it needs. Being ill creates a space. What do you choose to fill it with? Anxiety and despair or hope and self-compassion?

So slow down, take a breath and consider what direction you want to take. Remember that facing our vulnerability can give us immense strength.

If you're well right now and you have established a feeling of calm in your gut, continue to eat for diversity as much as you can. Try and give your old anxieties a good old hug from time to time. Mourn the take-out pizza, but make your own and celebrate the stuff you and your gut bugs can eat. This is about engaging in all elements of your gut healing journey, retraining your mind and microbes. If in doubt, touch your hands to your belly when you choose your food, sync into your self-care and self-love.

Healing is not an event. I'm deeply grateful to have my beautiful colon. I thank her each day for the works she does to keep me going. Yes, funny that she's a she, and well, whatever works for you. Go for it. Your journey may have begun before you read this book, but it won't end here. Know that the very act of reading this book is a step towards calming and healing your gorgeous gut. Keep journalling and talking your truth. Describe your symptoms and the impact they have on your life. When you are fully health articulate, you become your own best gut advocate.

This book is my offering to you as a fellow gut health traveller. I hope that you find in it the confidence to trust your gut. To learn to love the gift of the gut in your life. And the deep knowledge that you get to write the next chapter. You, dear one, get to choose how your gut story unfolds as you become the custodian of your microbiome; as you learn to tend to it and honour it, you'll start to see it as deeply connected to the wider global diversity of life on planet Earth.

And then you'll see your own journey is intimately interwoven, not just with your own beautiful bugs, but with the wider planet system too.

And, well, from this vantage point, those of us living with 'a troubled gut' become the outliers, the litmus test of a world where currently too little care is being taken to protect the diversity of our shared human biome. From this perspective, we're no longer the victims of IBD or IBS, but the *outliers* – the advocates for urgent change to the food industry and for protecting the environmental diversity of all parts of our beautiful planet, inner and outer.

*Be bold and brave*
*on your gut-loving journey.*

I wish you joy as you continue to live your very own authentic gut-led life.

# RESOURCES

## Part I: Gut Knowledge

Collen, A., 2015. *10% Human*. London: William Collins.

Enders, G., 2014, 2017. *Gut*. London: Scribe Publications.

Gottschall, E., 1994. *Breaking the Vicious Cycle*. New York: Kirkton Pr Ltd.

Greger, M., 2016. *How Not to Die*. London: Bluebird.

Jacka, F., 2019. *Brain Changer*. London: Yellow Kite.

Klein, D., 2013. *Self Healing: Colitis and Crohn's*. 4th ed. Maui: Living Nutrition Publications.

Korth, C.A., 2012. *The IBD Healing Plan and Recipe Book*. Alameda: Hunter House Inc.

Lukyanovsky, I., 2019. *Crohn's and Colitis Fix*. New York: Morgan James Publishing.

Mayer, E., 2018. *The Mind–Gut Connection*. New York: Harper Wave.

Mosley, M., 2017. *The Clever Guts Diet*. London: Short Books.

Spector, T., 2016. *The Diet Myth*. London: Weidenfeld & Nicholson.

### *Get to know your gut bugs*

Professor Tim Spectre has partnered with leading scientists using cutting-edge microbiome research to create www.joinzoe.com.

For more on the ethics of your food choices, explore www.slowfood.org.uk and www.navdanyainternational.org

For IBS, try the inspirational Happy Pear Cooking Course: www.happypearcourses.com

## Part II: Gut Compassion

Brach, T,. 2019. *Radical Compassion.* London: Rider.

Chödrön, P., 2001. *The Places That Scare You.* Boston: Shambhala.

Feldman Barrett, L., 2018. *How Emotions are Made.* London: Pan Macmillan.

Fogg, B.J., 2019. *Tiny Habits.* London: Ebury Publishing.

Griffin, S., 1999. *Made From This Earth.* London: Women's Press.

Hamilton, D., 2017. *The Five Side Effects of Kindness*. London: Hay House UK.

Holford, P., 2004. *New Optimum Nutrition Bible*. London: Piatkus Books Ltd.

Kline, N., 1999, *Time to Think.* London: Octopus.

Maté, G., 2019. *When the Body Says No.* London: Vermilion.

Morgan, K. and Watts, G., 2015. *The Coach's Casebook*. Cheltenham: Inspect & Adapt.

Mountain Dreamer, O., 1995. *The Invitation.* London: Thorsons.

Mosley, M., 2020. *Fast Asleep.* London: Short Books.

Neff, K., 2011. *Self-compassion.* New York: William Morrow.

Nhat Hanh, T., 1991. *Peace Is Every Step*. New York: Bantam Press.

Reading, S., 2017. *The Self-care Revolution.* London: Octopus.

Rolf Farrar, A., 2020. *The Wellfulness Project*. London: Aster.

Rucklidge, J. and Kaplan, B., 2021. *The Better Brain*. London: Vermilion.

Salzberg, S., 2002. *Loving Kindness*. Boston: Shambhala.

### *Social media and weblinks*

For the havening technique, a simple exercise to put you into a 'safe space' and reduce stress, look at www.havening.org.

For a brilliant yoga resource, check out www.yogawithadriene.com.

For building compassion – www.compassionatemind.co.uk or www.self-compassion.org (with Dr Kristin Neff).

For movement, take a look at the inspirational www.deepikamehta.in.

For one of the most inspiring new-generation gastroenterologists, follow @gut_love on Instagram with Dr Elena Ivanina.

Breathwork app: Wim Hof Method

Mindfulness app: Headspace

For post-surgery, check out @thebaglifeofbeck on Instagram.

For uplifting IBD discussion, follow @plentyandwellwithnat on Instagram.

For bloat-friendly inspiration, check out www.thetummydiaries.com (IBS).

## Part III: Gut Healing

Brown, B., 2015. *Daring Greatly.* London: Penguin Life.

Chopra, D., 1991. *Perfect Healing.* New York: Transworld Publishers Ltd.

Dethmer, J. and Chapman, D., 2015. *The 15 Commitments of Conscious Leadership.* Chicago: Dethmer, Chapman & Klemp.

Hamilton, D., 2015. *I Heart Me.* London: Hay House UK.

Harari, Y., 2014. *Sapiens.* London: Vintage.

Kay, A., 2018. *This Is Going to Hurt.* London: Picador.

Macchiochi, J., 2020. *Immunity.* London: Thorsons.

Murphy, K., 2019. *You're Not Listening.* London: Harvill Secker.

Perlmutter, D., 2016. *The Grain Brain Whole Life Plan.* London: Yellow Kite.

Perlmutter, D., 2015. *Brain Maker.* London: Yellow Kite.

Roth, G., 1999, 2008. *Sweat Your Prayers.* New York: M.H. Gill & Co.

Wall Kimmerer, R., 2020. *Braiding Sweetgrass.* London: Penguin Random House.

Ware, B., 2012. *The Top Five Regrets of the Dying.* Sydney: Hay House Australia.

### *Social media and weblinks*

For AID-IBD support: www.umassmed.edu/nutrition/ibd/ibdaid and the Facebook community: IBD-AID Diet Support.

For advice and food recommendations when following the low FODMAP diet, try the Monash University FODMAP Diet app.

For wider mental health support, look at charities Mind (www.mind.org.uk) or Samaritans (www.samaritans.org) in the UK.

National Alliance on Mental Illness (www.nami.org) in the USA .

For yoga and Ayurveda ideas, check out Ananta Ripa Ajmera (www.theancientway.co) or @ananta.one on Instagram.

A leading researcher on gut health is Dr Megan Rossi: @theguthealthdoctor on Instagram.

Gastroenterologist and plant-based advocate on Instagram: @dr.alandesmond.

Check out the handles @evekalinik and @thehappyguthut on Instagram.

## Part IV: Gut Integrity

Chödrön, P., 2001. *The Places That Scare You*. Boston: Shambhala.

Chödrön, P., 2002. *Comfortable with Uncertainty.* Boston: Shambala.

Coelho, P., 1998. *The Alchemist*. London: HarperCollins.

Goleman, D., 2003. *Healing Emotions*. Boston: Shambala

Grange, P., 2020. *Fear Less*. London: Vermilion.

Obama, M. 2018. *Becoming*. New York: Viking.

O'Donohue, J., 2003. *Divine Beauty.* London: Bantam Press.

Rogers, J, and Maini, A., 2016. *Coaching for Health*. Maidenhead: Open University Press.

### *Charities*

Crohn's and Colitis UK: www.crohnsandcolitis.org.uk

The Crohn's and Colitis Foundation (USA): www.crohnscolitisfoundation.org

IBS-specific charities include www.gutscharity.org.uk and www.theibsnetwork.org.

### *Podcasts*

Feel Better, Live More with Dr Rangan Chatterjee

Sounds True: Insights at the Edge with Tami Simon

### *Socia media and weblinks*

For all-round inspiration on the planetary gaia and gut health, check out Zach Bush.(www.zachbushmd.com) and the hashtag #breatheyourbiome.

## Part V: Gut-loving Food and Recipes

Chopra, D., 1991. *Perfect Healing*. New York: Transworld Publishers Ltd.

Desmond, A., 2021. *The Plant-Based Diet Revolution*. London: Yellow Kite.

Oliver, J., 2015. *Everyday Super Food*. London: Michael Joseph.

Wong, J., 2017. *How to Eat Better*. London: Octopus.

### *Grow your own*

For gardening inspiration, check out www.rekhagardenkitchen.com, @themontydon on Instagram, and Simplify Gardening and Self Sufficient Me on YouTube.

In the UK, check out www.seedcooperative.org.uk for gardening ideas.

### *Ethical brands*

Support your shopping and Gaia by choosing fair-trade products and companies with environmentally conscious business practices (www.ethicalconsumer.org). Of course, aim to buy from local producers, and I recommend the following family-based business in the UK:

Family-run organic and free-from foods: Amisa (www.amisa.co.uk)

Organic and fair-trade goods: Biona (www.biona.co.uk)

Raw and organic fermented food and drink: Loving Foods (www.lovingfoods.co.uk) – I'm loving their fermented kimchi right now! They are family-run and ethical.

Bespoke gut health advice and kefir: Chuckling Goat (www.chucklinggoat.co.uk)

Grains: Dove Organic flours and products (www.dovesfarm.co.uk)

Non-dairy milk: Lucy Bee (www.lucybee.com/collections/pantry), Plamil (www.plamilfoods.co.uk), Good Hemp (www.goodhemp.com) and Oatly (www.oatly.com)

Organic porridge oats: Flahavan's (www.flahavans.co.uk)

Healthy food at a click: Mindful Chef (www.mindfulchef.com) – we've tried these recipe boxes out as a treat, and they have great plant-based and ethically sourced options.

# REFERENCES


## About *Calm Your Gut*

1. NHS 24, 2016. 'Colostomy'. https://www.nhsinform.scot/tests-and-treatments/surgical-procedures/colostomy [Accessed April 2021]
2. Breines, J. et al., 2014. 'Self-compassion as a predictor of interleukin-6 response to acute psychosocial stress'. *Brain, Behavior, and Immunity*, 37:109–14. https://doi.org/10.1016/j.bbi.2013.11.006. Epub 2013 Nov 14. PMID: 24239953; PMCID: PMC4311753

## Part I: Gut Knowledge

1. M'Koma, A.E., 2013. 'Inflammatory bowel disease: an expanding global health problem'. *Clinical Medicine Insights: Gastroenterology*, 6:(3): 3–47. https://doi.org/10.4137/CGast.S12731
2. Caruso, R., Lo, B. and Núñez, G., 2020. 'Host–microbiota interactions in inflammatory bowel disease'. *Nature Reviews Immunology*, 20: 411–26. https://doi.org/10.1038/s41577-019-0268-7
3. Glassner, K. *et al.*, 2020. 'The microbiome and inflammatory bowel disease'. *The Journal of Allergy and Clinical Immunology*, 145(1):16–27. https://doi.org/10.1016/j.jaci.2019.11.003
4. Thomas, Z., 2020. 'Managing IBS at work: for sufferers and their employers'. https://www.posturite.co.uk/blog/managing-ibs-work-sufferers-employers [Accessed April 2021]
5. Nhat Hanh, T., 1991. *Peace Is Every Step*. New York: Bantam Press
6. Natasha Allergy Research Foundation, 2019. 'What is Natasha's Law?'. https://www.narf.org.uk/natashaslaw [Accessed April 2021]

7. Bush, Z., 2021. 'The last 30 years of microbiome research necessitates a radical shift in our model of human health'. Available at: www.zachbushmd.com/knowledge-virome [Accessed April 2021]
8. Glassner, K. *et al.*, 2020. 'The microbiome and inflammatory bowel disease'. *The Journal of Allergy and Clinical Immunology*, 145(1):16–27. https://doi.org/10.1016/j.jaci.2019.11.003
9. Geerlings, S. *et al.*, 2018. 'Akkermansia muciniphila in the human gastrointestinal tract: when, where, and how?' *Microorganisms*, 6(3):75. https://doi.org/10.3390/microorganisms6030075
10. NHS, 2018. 'Leaky-gut-syndrome'. https://www.nhs.uk/conditions/leaky-gut-syndrome/ [Accessed April 2021]
11. Collen, A., 2015. *10% Human*. London: William Collins, p64
12. Bonaz, B., Bazin, T. and Pellissier, S., 2018. 'The Vagus Nerve at the Interface of the Microbiota-Gut-Brain Axis'. *Frontiers in Neuroscience*, 12:49. https://doi.org/10.3389/fnins.2018.00049
13. Merton, T., 1972, 2007. *New Seeds of Contemplation (New Directions Paperbook)*. New York: New Directions
14. National Institute for Health and Care Excellence, 'Inflammatory bowel disease': https://www.nice.org.uk/guidance/conditions-and-diseases/digestive-tract-conditions/inflammatory-bowel-disease [Accessed April 2021]
15. Center for Applied Nutrition, https://www.umassmed.edu/nutrition/ [Accessed April 2021]
16. Lovelock, J., 2016. *Gaia*. Oxford: Oxford University Press
17. Collen, A., 2015. *10% Human*. London: William Collins, p64
18. Johnson, K., 2019. 'Gut microbiome composition and diversity are related to human personality traits'. *Human Microbiome Journal*, 15:100069. https://doi.org/10.1016/j.humic.2019.100069
19. Li, Y. *et al.*, 2014. 'Cesarean delivery and risk of inflammatory bowel disease: a systematic review and meta-analysis'. *Scandinavian Journal of Gastroenterology*, 49(7): 834–44. https://doi.org/10.3109/00365521.2014.910834. Epub 2014 Jun 18. PMID: 24940636
20. Derrien, M. Alvarez, A. and de Vos, W., 2019. 'The gut microbiota in the first decade of life'. *Trends in Microbiology*, 27(12):997–1010. https://doi.org/10.1016/j.tim.2019.08.001. Epub 2019 Aug 29. PMID: 31474424
21. Rutherford, A., 2016. 'The microbes in your body that you couldn't live without': https://www.bbc.com/future/article/20170321-why-your-diet-may-be-bad-for-your-gut-bacteria [Accessed April 2021]
22. Collen, A., 2015. *10% Human*. London: William Collins
23. Greger, M., 2016. *How Not to Die*. London: Bluebird
24. Nguyen, D. *et al.*, 2015. 'Formation and Degradation of Beta-casomorphins in Dairy Processing'. *Critical Reviews in Food Science and Nutrition*, 55(14): 1955–67. https://doi.org/10.1080/10408398.2012.740102

25. Berkman, E., 2018. 'Value-based choice: An integrative, neuroscience-informed model of health goals'. *Psychology and Health*, 33(1): 40–57. https://doi.org/10.1080/08870446.2017.1316847

26. Jewell, T., 2019. 'What causes dysbiosis and how is it treated?'. www.healthline.com/health/digestive-health/dysbiosis [Accessed April 2021]

27. Morris, G. *et al.*, 2016. 'The role of microbiota and intestinal permeability in the pathophysiology of autoimmune and neuroimmune processes with an emphasis on inflammatory bowel disease, type 1 diabetes and chronic fatigue syndrome'. *Current Pharmaceutical Design*, 22(40): 6058–75. https://pubmed.ncbi.nlm.nih.gov/27634186/

28. Carding, S. *et al.*, 2015. 'Dysbiosis of the gut microbiota in disease'. *Microbial Ecology in Health and Disease*, 2;26: 2619. doi: 10.3402/mehd.v26.26191

29. O'Doherty, K.C. *et al*, 2014. 'Opinion: Conservation and stewardship of the human microbiome'. *Proceedings of the National Academy of Sciences of the United States of America*, 111(40):14312-14313. https://doi.org/10.1073/pnas.1413200111

30. Glassner, K. *et al.*, 2020. 'The microbiome and inflammatory bowel disease'. *The Journal of Allergy and Clinical Immunology*, 145(1):16–27. https://doi.org/10.1016/j.jaci.2019.11.003

31. Stewart, L., 2020. '5 Gut Bacteria with unusual Health Benefits'. https://atlasbiomed.com/blog/top-5-gut-bacteria-with-unusual-health-benefits/ [Accessed April 2021]

32. Mosley, M., 2017. *The Clever Guts Diet*. London: Short Books, p56

33. Glassner, K. *et al.*, 2020. 'The microbiome and inflammatory bowel disease'. *The Journal of Allergy and Clinical Immunology*, 145(1):16–27. https://doi.org/10.1016/j.jaci.2019.11.003


## Part II: Gut Compassion


1. Dingham, M., 2014. 'Know Your Brain: Amygdala': https://www.neuroscientificallychallenged.com/blog/know-your-brain-amygdala [Accessed April 2021]

2. Breines, J. et al., 2014. 'Self-compassion as a predictor of interleukin-6 response to acute psychosocial stress'. *Brain, Behavior, and Immunity*, 37:109–14. https://doi.org/10.1016/j.bbi.2013.11.006. Epub 2013 Nov 14. PMID: 24239953; PMCID: PMC4311753

3. Nguyen, T. *et al.*, 2021. 'Association of loneliness and wisdom with gut microbial diversity and composition: An exploratory study'. *Frontiers in Psychiatry*. https://doi.org/10.3389/fpsyt.2021.648475

4. Jacka, F., 2019. *Brain Changer*. London: Yellow Kite, p107

5. The Hearty Soul, 2020. '6 Ways to Instantly Stimulate Your Vagus Nerve to Relieve Inflammation'. https://www.iahe.com/docs/articles/6_Ways_to_

Instantly_Stimulate_Your_Vagus_Nerve_to_Relieve_Inflammation.pdf [Accessed April 2021]

6. Feldman Barrett, L., 2018. *How Emotions are Made*. London: Pan Macmillan
7. Jacka, F., 2019. *Brain Changer*. London: Yellow Kite, p62–67
8. Rucklidge, J. and Kaplan, B., 2021. *The Better Brain*. London: Vermilion
9. Jiango, L., 2019. 'Altered gut metabolome contributes to depression-like behaviors in rats exposed to chronic unpredictable mild stress'. *Translational Psychiatry*, 9:40. https://www.nature.com/articles/s41398-019-0391-z
10. University of Birmingham, 2020. 'Microbiome Treatment Centre' https://www.birmingham.ac.uk/university/colleges/mds/facilities/advanced-therapies-facility/microbiome-treatment-centre.aspx [Accessed April 2021]
11. González-Arancibia C, *et al.*, 2019. 'Do your gut microbes affect your brain dopamine?' *Psychopharmacology*, 236: 1611–22. https://doi.org/10.1007/s00213-019-05265-5
12. Jacka, F., 2019. *Brain Changer*. London: Yellow Kite, p115
13. Maté, G., 2019. *When the Body Says No*. London: Vermilion, p137–139; Drossman, D.A. (1998), 'Presidential Address: Gastrointestinal Illness and the Biopsychosocial model,' *Psychosomatic Medicine 60*, pp258–67
14. Chevalier, G. *et al.*, 2012. 'Earthing: health implications of reconnecting the human body to the earth's surface electrons'. *Journal of Environmental and Public Health*, 2012:291541. https://doi.org/10.1155/2012/291541
15. Panhwar, M. *et al.*, 2019. 'Risk of myocardial infarction in inflammatory bowel disease: a population-based national study'. *Inflammatory Bowel Diseases*, 25(6):1080-1087. doi: 10.1093/ibd/izy354. PMID: 30500938
16. MacKenzie, D., 2019. 'We may finally know what causes Alzheimer's – and how to stop it'. https://www.newscientist.com/article/2191814-we-may-finally-know-what-causes-alzheimers-and-how-to-stop-it/#ixzz6sZsgczcN [Accessed April 2021]
17. Hamilton, D., 2017. *The Five Side Effects of Kindness*. London: Hay House UK
18. Junker, Y. *et al.*, 2017. 'Wheat amylase trypsin inhibitors drive intestinal inflammation via activation of toll-like receptor 4'. *Journal of Experimental Medicine*, 209(13):2395–408. https://doi.org/10.1084/jem.20102660
19. BBC News, 2011. Chorleywood: The bread that changed Britain'. www.bbc.co.uk/news/magazine-13670278 [Accessed April 2021]
20. Langdon, A., Crook, N. and Dantast, G., 2016. 'The effects of antibiotics on the microbiome throughout development and alternative approaches for therapeutic modulation'. *Genome Medicine*, 8: 39. doi: 10.1186/s13073-016-0294-z
21. Stoll, J., 2021. 'Eating meals while watching TV in the UK in 2019/2020, by age group'. https://www.statista.com/statistics/1127324/eating-meals-while-watching-tv-uk-age-group/ [Accessed April 2021]

22. Aviva, 2017. 'Sleepless cities revealed as one in three adults suffer from insomnia'. https://www.aviva.com/newsroom/news-releases/2017/10/Sleepless-cities-revealed-as-one-in-three-adults-suffer-from-insomnia/ [Accessed April 2021]

23. Smith, R.P. *et al.*, 2019. 'Gut microbiome diversity is associated with sleep physiology in humans'. *PLoS ONE*, 14(10):e0222394. https://doi.org/10.1371/journal.pone.0222394

24. Hartl, G., 2001. 'The World Health Report 2001: Mental Disorders affect one in four'. https://www.who.int/news/item/28-09-2001-the-world-health-report-2001-mental-disorders-affect-one-in-four-people [Accessed April 2021]

25. Gazibegovic, N., 2019. 'How do different colours affect your mood, judgement and physiology?'. https://blogs.unimelb.edu.au/sciencecommunication/2018/10/09/how-do-different-colours-affect-your-mood-judgement-and-physiology/ [Accessed April 2021]

26. Drake, N., 2019. 'Our nights are getting brighter, and Earth is paying the price'. https://www.nationalgeographic.com/science/article/nights-are-getting-brighter-earth-paying-the-price-light-pollution-dark-skies [Accessed April 2021]

27. Smith R.P. *et al.*, 2019. 'Gut microbiome diversity is associated with sleep physiology in humans'. *PLoS ONE*, 14(10):e0222394. https://doi.org/10.1371/journal.pone.0222394

28. Mosley, M., 2017. *The Clever Guts Diet.* London: Short Books, p142

29. Li, Y. *et al.*, 2018. 'The role of microbiome in insomnia, circadian disturbance and depression'. *Frontiers of Psychiatry*, 9: 669. https://doi.org/10.3389/fpsyt.2018.00669

30. Robert, S., 2020. 'Can't sleep? Prebiotics could help'. https://www.sciencedaily.com/releases/2020/03/200303155658.htm [Accessed April 2021]

31. Cameron, J., 2020. *The Artist's Way.* London: Souvenir Press

32. Sokal, K. and Sokal, P., 2011. 'Earthing the human body influences physiologic processes'. *Journal of Alternative and Complementary Medicine*, 17(4): 301–8. doi: 10.1089/acm.2010.0687

33. Kim, S. *et al.*, 2016. 'Effects of aromatherapy on menopausal symptoms, perceived stress and depression in middle-aged women: a systematic review'. *Journal of Korean Academy of Nursing*, 46(5):619–29. https://doi.org/10.4040/jkan.2016.46.5.619

34. Takagi, C. *et al.*, 2019. 'Evaluating the effect of aromatherapy on a stress marker in healthy subjects'. *Journal of Pharmaceutical Health Care and Sciences,* 5: 18. https://doi.org/10.1186/s40780-019-0148-0

35. Lee, Y., 2011. 'A systematic review on the anxiolytic effects of aromatherapy in people with anxiety symptoms'. *Journal of Alternative and Complementary Medicine*, 17(2): 101–8. https://doi.org/10.1089/acm.2009.0277

## Part III: Gut Healing


1. Gould, D., 2019. 'Introducing biodiversity: the intersection of taste & sustainability'. https://foodtechconnect.com/2019/01/07/biodiverse-food-intersection-taste-sustainability/ [Accessed April 2021]
2. Shiva, V. and Singh, V., 2017. 'HEALTH PER ACRE Organic Solutions to Hunger and Malnutrition'. https://navdanyainternational.org/wp-content/uploads/2017/07/Health-Per-Acre.pdf [Accessed April 2021]
3. Haskey, N. and Gibson, D., 2017. 'An examination of diet for the maintenance of remission in inflammatory bowel disease', *Nutrients*. 9(3):259. https://doi.org/10.3390/nu9030259
4. Dowd, A.J. and Jung, M., 2017. 'Self-compassion directly and indirectly predicts dietary adherence and quality of life among adults with celiac disease'. *Appetite*, 113: 293–300. doi: 10.1016/j.appet.2017.02.023. Epub 2017 Feb 20
5. Jeavans, C., 2014. 'How much sugar do we eat?'. www.bbc.co.uk/news/health-27941325 [Accessed April 2021]
6. Coughlan, M., 2015. 'Could emulsifiers in food damage the gut?'. www.weforum.org/agenda/2015/04/could-emulsifiers-in-food-damage-the-gut [Accessed April 2021]
7. Rossi, M., 2017, 'A Beginner's Guide to the Low-FODMAP Diet'. www.healthline.com/nutrition/low-fodmap-diet [Accessed April 2021]
8. Chopra, D., 1991. *Perfect Healing*. New York: Transworld Publishers Ltd
9. Rauf, D., 2020. 'The Mediterranean Diet May Cut the Risk of One Type of Inflammatory Bowel Disease'. https://www.everydayhealth.com/crohns-disease/mediterranean-diet-may-cut-risk-of-one-type-of-inflammatory-bowel-disease/ [Accessed April 2021]
10. Center for Applied Nutrition, 'Sample daily menus for each phase'. https://www.umassmed.edu/nutrition/ibd/sample-daily-menus-for-each-phase/ [Accessed April 2021]
11. Albrecht, P., Banaszkiewicz, A. and Albrecht, P., 2015. 'The role of dietary fibre in inflammatory bowel disease', *Przegląd Gastroenterologiczny,* 3(3):135–41. doi: 10.5114/pg.2015.52753
12. Salim, S. *et al.*, 2013. 'Air pollution effects on the gut microbiota: a link between exposure and inflammatory disease'. *Gut Microbes*, 5(2):215–9. doi: https://doi.org/10.4161/gmic.27251. Epub 2013 Dec 20
13. Wall Kimmerer, R., 2020. *Braiding Sweetgrass*. London: Penguin Random House, p236
14. Henriques, M., 2019. 'Is it worth taking probiotics after antibiotics?': https://www.bbc.com/future/article/20190124-is-it-worth-taking-probiotics-after-antibiotics [Accessed April 2021]
15. Shen, Z. *et al.*, 2018. 'Relationship between intestinal microbiota and ulcerative colitis: Mechanisms and clinical application of probiotics and

fecal microbiota transplantation'. *World Journal of Gastroenterology*, 24(1): 5–14. doi: 10.3748/wjg.v24.i1.5

16. Richardson, R., 2017. 'What You Should Eat During and After Antibiotics'. https://www.healthline.com/nutrition/what-to-eat-antibiotics [Accessed April 2021]
17. Kleessen, B. *et al.*, 2007. 'Jerusalem artichoke and chicory inulin in bakery products affect faecal microbiota of healthy volunteers'. *British Journal of Nutrition*, 98(3): 540–9. doi: 10.1017/S0007114507730751. Epub 2007 Apr 20
18. Salvin, J., 2013. 'Fiber and prebiotics: mechanisms and health benefits'. *Nutrients*, 5(4): 1417–35. https://doi.org/10.3390/nu5041417
19. González-Castejón, M., Visioli, F. and Rodriguez-Casado, A., 2012. 'Diverse biological activities of dandelion'. *Nutrition Reviews*, 70;9, 534–47, https://doi.org/10.1111/j.1753-4887.2012.00509.x
20. Harari, Y., 2014. *Sapiens*. London: Vintage
21. Jacka, F., 2019. *Brain Changer*. London: Yellow Kite, p63
22. Chang, E. and Dolan, K., 2016. 'Diet, gut microbes, and the pathogenesis of inflammatory bowel diseases'. *Molecular Nutrition and Food Research*, 61(1):10.1002/mnfr.201600129. https://doi.org/10.1002/mnfr.201600129. Epub 2016 Aug 15
23. Lie, M. *et al.*, 2018. 'Low dose Naltrexone for induction of remission in inflammatory bowel disease patients'. *Journal of Translational Medicine*, 16(1):55. https://doi.org/10.1186/s12967-018-1427-5
24. Roland, J., 2019. 'Is CBD a safe and effective form of treatment for IBD, and what form to use it?'. https://www.healthline.com/health/cbd-for-ibd [Accessed April 2021]
25. Harvard Health Publishing, 2019. 'Time-sensitive-clues-about-cardiovascular-risk'. https://www.health.harvard.edu/heart-health/time-sensitive-clues-about-cardiovascular-risk [Accessed April 2021]
26. Ware, B., 2012. *The Top Five Regrets of the Dying*. Sydney: Hay House Australia
27. Nguyen, T. *et al.*, 2021. 'Association of loneliness and wisdom with gut microbial diversity and composition: an exploratory study.' *Frontiers in Psychiatry*: https://doi.org/10.3389/fpsyt.2021.648475
28. Roth, G., 1999. *Sweat Your Prayers*. New York: M.H. Gill & Co
29. Engels M., Cross, R.K. and Long, M., 2017. 'Exercise in patients with inflammatory bowel diseases: current perspectives'. *Clin Exp Gastroenterol*, 11:1–11. https://doi.org/10.2147/CEG.S120816. eCollection 2018
30. StopColonCancerNow.com, 'Exercise'. www.stopcoloncancernow.com/colon-cancer-prevention/prevention/exercise [Accessed April 2021]
31. Stelter, G., 2018. 'Yoga Poses for IBS'. https://www.healthline.com/health/yoga-poses-for-ibs [Accessed April 2021]
32. *Ibid.*

## Part IV: Gut Integrity

1. Rohn, J., 1996. *Leading an Inspired Life*. Nightingale Conant
2. De Bellefonds, C., 2020. 'What men should know about Crohn's disease': www.everydayhealth.com/crohns-disease/how-crohns-affects-men [Accessed April 2021]
3. Kim, N. and Kim, Y., 2018. 'Sex-gender differences in irritable bowel syndrome'. *Journal of Neurogastroenterology and Motility*, 24(4): 544–58. https://doi.org/10.5056/jnm18082
4. Bernstein, M. *et al.*, 2012. 'Gastrointestinal symptoms before and during menses in women with IBD'. *Alimentary Pharmacology and Therapeutics*, 36:135–44. https://doi.org/10.1111/j.1365-2036.2012.05155.x
5. Cumberlege, J., 2020. 'First Do No Harm'. https://www.immdsreview.org.uk/downloads/IMMDSReview_Web.pdf [Accessed April 2021]
6. Haskell, H., 2020. 'Cumberlege review exposes stubborn and dangerous flaws in healthcare'. *BMJ*, 370:m3099. https://doi.org/10.1136/bmj.m3099
7. Newman, T., 2017. 'Is the Placebo Effect Real?': https://www.medicalnewstoday.com/articles/306437 [Accessed April 2021]
8. Dragon, N., 2018. 'New colon and rectal cancer screening guidelines'. https://intermountainhealthcare.org/blogs/topics/transforming-healthcare/2018/06/new-colon-and-rectal-cancer-screening-guidelines/ [Accessed April 2021]
9. Zimmer, K., 2019. 'There's a troubling rise in colorectal cancer among young adults'. https://www.the-scientist.com/news-opinion/theres-a-troubling-rise-in-colorectal-cancer-among-young-adults--66354 [Accessed April 2021]
10. Jalanka, J. *et al.*, 2015. 'Effects of bowel cleansing on the intestinal microbiota'. *Gut*, 4(10):1562–8. https://gut.bmj.com/content/64/10/1562. Epub 2014 Dec 19. PMID: 25527456
11. Powell, A., 2018. 'Researchers study how it seems to change the brain in depressed patients'. https://news.harvard.edu/gazette/story/2018/04/harvard-researchers-study-how-mindfulness-may-change-the-brain-in-depressed-patients/ [Accessed April 2021]
12. Coelho, P., 1998. *The Alchemist*. London: HarperCollins

## Part V: Gut-loving Food and Recipes

1. Perlmutter, D., 2016. *The Grain Brain Whole Life Plan*. London: Yellow Kite
2. Oliver, J., 2015. *Everyday Super Food*. London: Michael Joseph, p292
3. Wong, J., 2017. *How to Eat Better*. London: Octopus, p90

# ACKNOWLEDGEMENTS

I'm grateful to the little gang of first readers for their patience: Tina, Marie, Sean and Gerardine. To Sarajane Aris for her mentorship, which supported me to honour my gut and my creative longings.

To Emily Arbis, my editor at Hay House. Thanks to the wider Hay House team for their faith and generosity: Michelle Pilley, Susie Bertinshaw, Lizzi Marshall, Portia Chauhan, Jo Burgess, Katherine O'Brien, Sandy Draper and Tom Cole. And well, if you feel you've got a story to tell, head along to a Hay House Writer's Workshop – you never quite know what will come of it!

To all the Psychologies team for championing growth mindset in an online community of inspiring women that I'm proud to contribute to, with an extra special mention to Suzy Walker and Ali Roff-Farrar.

To Kim Morgan and all the Barefoot team for the inspirational journey we have been on together. I appreciate the power of every coaching conversation I have had with each one of you! To Shirzad for creating the Positive Intelligence programme and my fellow coaches, James, Peta and Urvashi, for your bravery and openness in the process. To Polly and the Writers Readers Group for many fun evenings chatting about writing in all its many forms.

Thank you to the many other folk too numerous to mention (you know who you are – Ed, you feature here a lot!), who have listened to me talk about our gut bugs with humour and interest. To Pete Mosley for your calm, considered advice when I most needed it. To Leddra Chapman for your insight and knowledge, and to Bridgeen Duffy for simply being all-round brilliant. To my fellow Chucklers for your generosity and support.

To Marketa, Hannah and my fellow Goddesses at The Tree of Life, for holding a space of sacred connection. To Ru for being the caretaker of the allotment and a great uncle to Isla Mae.

I want to give special mention to the NHS staff: my consultant, nurses, doctors, orderlies and chaplains, who treated me with such kindness and care in my moment of health crisis. You do precious work every day. Thank you for retaining your humanity and compassion even in such challenging times.

This book is shaped by many conversations with courageous and inspirational individuals from the IBD tribe and IBS community who shared their stories: some are funny and fascinating, some about surgery at a young age are simply heart-rending. It's been an honour to witness how many of us are starting to talk more openly about our gorgeous guts.

Finally, to my beloved husband, David, for supporting me! Put simply, your kindness and generosity light up my life.

# INDEX


**A**

adrenaline 17, 18
affirmations 151, 196
  breathe out gut-loving affirmations 151–2
Akkermansia 57
alcohol 39, 99, 134–5, 148
allergic responses 13–14
alternative medicine 192–3, 202–3
amylase 6, 90
anaphylaxis 13
anti-inflammatory lifestyle 135–6
antibiotics 38–9, 89, 136–7
anxiety 63–7
  anxious gut reflection 73–4
  and food 67, 75, 87
  improving vagal tone 65–6
  and shame 70
  and sleep 98–100
  *see also* mental health; stress
apple cider vinegar 141
appointments 199–202
aromatherapy 103–5
artificial sweeteners 120
autoimmune reactions 13–15
Ayurvedic medicine 125–6, 142, 225

**B**

Bacteroidetes 56, 98
Barnesiella 57
base belly breathing 30–32
bedroom environment 96–7
belly massage 103–7
Belly Metta Bhavana practice 79–80
bifidobacteria 56, 83, 98, 138–9
bisphenol A 135
bloating 24, 55–6, 156, 160
BMI 129
the brain
  and food 48–9
  and inflammation 76–7, 98
  and stress 17, 63, 210
  vagus nerve connection to the gut 13, 16–17, 18
brain fog 44, 133
bread 87–8, 249–50
breakfast 229–35
breathing practices 152–6
  base belly breathing *30*, 30–32
  breathe out gut-loving affirmations 151–2
  importance of 29, 32
  when flaring 147

bromelain 85
broth 148
brunches 229–42
butyrate 56–7
butyric acid 84

## C

cancer 11, 166, 194
cannabidiol (CBD) 149
carbohydrates 89, 120, 127–8
carminative herbs 99, 257
casomorphin 44, 48
chakras 161, 213
- base belly breathing *30*, 30–32
- and dance 173–4
- gut-healing visualization 162–3
- the Gut Love Dance 174–8
- and yoga 167

cheese 44, 48
chemicals, exposure to 15–16, 88, 119, 135–6
chewing, importance of 6, 35, 90, 218
chocolate 140
chronic inflammation 14–16, *15*
- cycle of *34*

chyme 7
cloves 140, 257
collagen powder 147–8
colon *6*, 8, *33*, 34
colonoscopies 194–7
communicating needs 187–91, 199–202
compassion *see* self-compassion
complementary medicine 192–3, 202–3
coriander 257
cortisol 17, 18, 66, 95, 161
Crohn's disease (CD) 10–12, 105–7, 148
cycling 171

## D

dairy products 44, 48, 124, 130
dancing 173–80
- aligning head, heart & gut 178–80
- the Gut Love Dance 174–8
- tree dancing 171–2

depression and diet 67–9, 103
- *see also* mental health

desserts & treats 254–7
diet(s) 115–18
- changing slowly 210–12
- eliminate with love 143–4
- elimination diets 76–8, 116, 118–21
- fad diets 129–30
- fasting 132
- and flares 147–9
- and inflammation 14–16, *34*, 44–5, 67–9
- medical opinion 129–30
- and microbiome 15–16
- plant-based 126–7
- Western 16, 28, 116, 142–3

the digestive system *6*, 6–8, *33*
- Gut Gaia visualization 35–7
- through a lifespan 37–41

disaccharides 124
doctors 192–3, 199–202
- medical opinion and diets 129–30
- relationship with patients 187–8, 190–92, 199–202

dopamine 44, 48, 68
drinks 99, 257–8
duodenum 7, *33*, 34
dysbiosis 44–5
- planning response to 134–8

## E

eating
- being present with your plate 92
- eating out 205–6

during flares 147
mindful practices 90–93
and stress 17–18, 87
elimination diets 76–8, 118–21, 123–30
eliminate with love 143–4
emotions 63, 163–4
anxious gut reflection 73–4
Belly Metta Bhavana practice 79–80
reframing responses to 66
*see also* anxiety; self-compassion; stress
emulsifiers 121
endoscopies 196–7
endotoxins 14, *34*
environment 15–16, 41, 136
enzymes 6, 90
epigenetics 41
exercise 165–6
during flares 148
yoga 166–70
exercises
30-day love your belly challenge 216–19
anxious gut reflection 73–4
base belly breathing *30*, 30–32
being present with your plate 92
Belly Metta Bhavana practice 79–80
breathe out gut-loving affirmations 151–2
cat/cow 101, 168
child's pose 170
corpse pose 102–3
eliminate with love 143–4
family foods 47–8
flare reflection 150
food iceberg 48–9
get to know your gut story 38–41
Gut Gaia visualization 35–7
gut-healing visualization 162–3
gut health vision 52
gut life letter 58
the Gut Love Dance 174–8
gut love massage 105–7
gut-loving foot massage *108*, 108–9
gut network review 203
gut reflecting 159, 200
gut vision board 216
intuitive eating guide 86
knees to chest 169–70
learning gut compassion 71–3
a love letter from your gut 109–10, 215
mindful gut-care practice 153–4
reclining twist 168
roadmap to gut integrity 213–14
warrior pose II 168–9
your f**k it motivation maker 78

**F**

family foods 47–8
family life 204–7
fasting 132
fats 121, 132
fennel seeds 156, 258
fermented foods 83, 98, 138–9, 141, 252–4
fibre 131, 141
fight or flight response 17, 63
flares 145–6
and colonoscopies 195
and dancing 173–80
and diet 147–9
and exercise 165–6
flare reflection 150
gut-healing visualization 162–3
healing 147–50, 160–64
and journalling 150–51, 157–8
and mindful movement 171–2
and mindful practices 150–56, 161–4
planning for 134–7
and yoga 166–70

food 226–7
addiction to 44–5, 68, 89, 119, 120
being present with your plate 92
family foods 47–8
fermented 83, 98, 138–9, 141, 252–4
and flares 147–9
food iceberg 48–9
free-from products 130
growing 228–9
gut-healing 131–4
high-sugar 44–5
importance of diversity 116–18
intuitive eating guide 86
and mental health 67
the mindful food flow principle 84–6
natural instincts for 83–7, 89–90
organic 131–2, 228–9
processed *see* processed food
psychology of 44–6
relationship with 47–9, 75
shopping 85–7, 116–17
and sleep 98–9
treats 207
trigger foods *see* trigger foods
*see also* diet(s); eating
food allergies 13–14
food combining 125–6
food diaries 132–4, 147
food mood trackers 132–4
food values 46–7
foot care 107–9
gut-loving foot massage *108*, 108–9
free-from products 130
fruit & vegetables 131, 228–9

**G**

Gaia hypothesis 32–3
and the gut 32–7, 116
Gut Gaia visualization 35–7
gardening 131, 172, 228–9
gastritis 15
gender and gut health 188–9, 190–91
ginger 258
gluten 87–8
gluten-free diets 28, 118, 130
goal setting 51–8
grace 91–3
grains 87–8
green tea 139
gut
lining/wall 14–16, *15*
and stress 16–19
through a lifespan 37–41
*see also* microbiome
gut instincts 83–7, 89–90

**H**

habits, changing 51–4, 210–12
by reframing 66
your f**k it motivation maker 78
healing 214–15
*see also* diet(s); mindful practices
health *see* mental health; physical health
health professionals *see* doctors
the heart and inflammation 76–7
herbs 99, 140, 156, 228, 257
hydrating 147–8

**I**

IBD Anti-inflammatory Diet (IBD-AID) 128–9
IBD (inflammatory bowel disease) 3, 10–12
and diet 28
and mindful practices 29–32
and physical health 76–7
treatments 11, 67, 192–3
*see also* flares

IBS (irritable bowel syndrome) 3, 9–10
  and diet 124–5
  gut love massage 105–7
  and women 190
  *see also* flares
ileum 7
Immunoglobulin E response (IgE) 13
Immunoglobulin G response (IgG) 14
inflammation 10–11, 12–14
  chronic 14–16, *15*, *34*
  and diet 14–16, *34*, 44–5, 67–9
  and health 76–7
  postprandial 132
  and sleep 95–6
intestinal permeability 14, *15*
intestines
  large 8, *33*, 34
  small 7–8, *33*, 34
intuitive eating guide 86

**J**
jejunum 7
journalling 19, 70
  anxious gut reflection 73–4
  bedtime routine 99
  benefits of 157–8
  flare reflection 150
  food iceberg 48–9
  food mood trackers 132–4
  get to know your gut story 38–41
  gut Gaia visualization 35–7
  gut health vision 52
  gut life letter 58
  gut network review 203
  gut reflecting 159, 200
  a love letter from your gut 109–10, 215
  and movement 180
  reflection 181
  your f**k it motivation maker 78
junk food *see* processed food

**K**
kefir 138
kimchi 139
kindness 81
  *see also* self-compassion
kitchen environment 225–6
knowledge *see* self-knowledge

**L**
lactobacillus 55–6, 83, 138–9
language and communicating needs 187–91
large intestine 8, *33*, 34
leaky gut 14–16, *15*, 147–9
lifespan and the digestive system 37–41
lifestyle 15–16, 41, 135–6
  *see also* stress
Lovelock, James 32–3
low dose naltrexone (LDN) 149
low FODMAP diet 56, 124–5, 227–8

**M**
main meals 243–9
mantras: Belly Metta Bhavana practice 79–80
massage
  gut love massage 105–7
  gut-loving foot massage *108*, 108–9
  and sleep 103–7
massage oil 104–5
meat 127
medicine *see* alternative medicine; Western medicine
Mediterranean diet 127
men and gut health 188–90
mental health
  and food 67
  and microbiome 38, 56, 64, 67–9
  *see also* stress

microbiome 8, 9
and diet 15–16
and dysbiosis 44–5
and environment 16, 41, 136
good bacteria 55–7
importance of 37–8
and mental health 38, 56, 64, 67–9
and personal history 38–41
and physical health 54–6
resilience of 137–8
uniqueness of 117–18
milk 257–8
mind and body *see* vagus nerve
mindful food flow principle 84–6
mindful practices 151–6, 161–4
being present with your plate 92
breathe out gut-loving affirmations 151–2
cat/cow yoga 101
eating 90–93
and IBD 29–32
micro-moments 155–6
mindful gut-care practice 153–4
mindful movement 171–2
shopping 85–7
and sleep 100–101
*see also* breathing practices
monosaccharides 124
motivation 77–9
your f**k it motivation maker 78
movement
exercise 148, 165–70
mindful movement 171–2

**N**
nature, calming influence of 101–3
NCGS (non-coeliac gluten sensitivity) 88
nervous system 17, 18, 29–32
networking *see* support networks
non-coeliac gluten sensitivity (NCGS) 88
nutmeg 257

**O**
oesophagus 7
oil
massage oil 104–5
olive oil 84, 132, 141
oligosaccharides 124
olive oil 84, 132, 141
omega-rich food 141–2
oral hygiene 136
organic food 131–2
orthorexia 75–6
ostomies 11–12

**P**
parasympathetic nervous system 17, 18
importance of breathing 29–32
patients
communicating needs 187–91, 199–202
gender differences 188–91
relationship with doctors 187–8, 190–92, 199–202
*see also* support networks
pelvic floor 167
peristalsis 7, 8
pharmanutrition 140–42
physical health 54–6
pineapple 85
plant-based diets 126–7
pollution 135
polyols 124
polyphenols 134–5, 139–40
postprandial inflammation 132
prebiotics 98, 128, 137, 139
probiotics 55–6, 98, 128, 137, 138–9
processed food 14, *34*, 67–9, 84
elimination diets 76–8, 118–21, 123–30
grain products 87–9
and gut dysbiosis 44–5
psychology of food 44–6

**Q**

Qigong 171
questionnaire 20–26

**R**

recipes
  autumn aches 236
  banana, cacao and vanilla ice cream 256–7
  easy breakfast porridge 231–2
  easy sauerkraut 252–3
  fermented cucumber 253–4
  fresh summer soup 237–9
  gut-loving simple salad dressing 241
  homemade oatcakes 251
  lentil dhal 243–5
  pancake heaven 233–5
  simple homemade bread 249–50
  spring simple super green (smoothie) 235–6
  Spring/Summer Falafel with Guacamole and Lentil Flatbreads 247–9
  summer bircher muesli 230–31
  summer smoothie 236
  tasty treat flapjacks 254–5
  vegan bolognese 245–7
  warming autumnal salad 241–2
  warming root veg soup 239–40
  weekend brunch 232–3
  winter fill me up 237
refined carbohydrates 89, 120, 127–8
reflexology 107–9, *108*
relationships 158–9, 204–7
resilience, building up 137–8
root chakra
  base belly breathing *30*, 30–32
  gut-healing visualization 162–3
  and yoga 167
Roseburia 57

**S**

salads 241–2
sauerkraut 139
self-awareness 210–12
self-compassion 70–74
  anxious gut reflection 73–4
  Belly Metta Bhavana practice 79–80
  and diet 76–8, 118–21
  flare reflection 150
  and healing 64–6, 70–74
  learning gut compassion 71–3
  when flaring 149, 160
  your f**k it motivation maker 78
  *see also* mindful practices
self-knowledge
  base belly breathing 31–2
  breathing with awareness 30–31
  Gut Gaia visualization 32–7
  journalling 19
  recognising triggers/early warning signs 29–30
  your gut story 37–41
serotonin 68
shame, transforming 70–74
shopping 85–7, 116–17, 204
sleep 101
  bedroom environment 96–7
  bedtime drinks 99
  calming routines 99–100
  cat/cow yoga 101
  corpse pose 102–3
  and diet 98–9
  during flares 148
  foot care 107–9
  gut love massage 105–7
  importance of 95–6
  improving 97–110
  massage routines 103–7
  mindful practices 100–101
  nature as a calming influence 101–3
sleep hygiene 96–7

small intestine 7–8, *33*, 34
smoothies 235–7
solar plexus chakra 161, 213
  base belly breathing *30*, 30–32
  gut-healing visualization 162–3
soup 237–40
Specific Carbohydrate Diet (SCD) 127–8
spices 257–8
steroids 192–3
stomach 7
  belly massage 103–7
  Belly Metta Bhavana practice 79–80
stress 155, 160–62
  and eating 17–18, 87
  and the gut 16–19
  improving vagal tone 65–6
  and inflammation 64, 69
  learning gut compassion 71–3
  and sleep 99–100
  triggers 19
  *see also* mindful practices
sugar
  dangers of 17, 44–5, 98
  reducing 120
supplements 139, 149
support networks 145–6, 157–9, 204–7
  gut network review 203
  *see also* doctors
sympathetic nervous system 17

**T**
treatments 11, 67, 192–3
  colonoscopies 194–7
treats 207
tree dancing 171–2
trigger foods 44–5, 49, 129
  avoiding 76–8, 119
  food diaries 132–4
  *see also* elimination diets
turmeric 258

**U**
ulcerative colitis (UC) 10–12
  gut love massage 105–7

**V**
vagal tone 64–6
vagus nerve 13, 16–17, 18
  and dancing 178–80
  and foot massage 109
  importance of breathing 29–32
vegan diets 126–7
vegetables 131, 228–9
villi 7–8, *34*
vision boards 215–16
visualizations
  Gut Gaia visualization 35–7
  gut-healing visualization 162–3

**W**
walking 171
water 136, 147–8
Western diet 16, 28, 116, 142–3
  *see also* processed food
Western lifestyle 15–16, 41
  *see also* stress
Western medicine 192–3, 199–202
wheat 87–8
whole foods 132
wine 134–5
women
  and gut health 188, 190
  and IBS 190
worry *see* anxiety

**Y**
yoga 166–70
  cat/cow 101, 168
  child's pose 170
  corpse pose 102–3
  knees to chest 169–70
  reclining twist 168
  warrior pose II 168–9
yoghurt, live 139

# ABOUT THE AUTHOR

David Busst

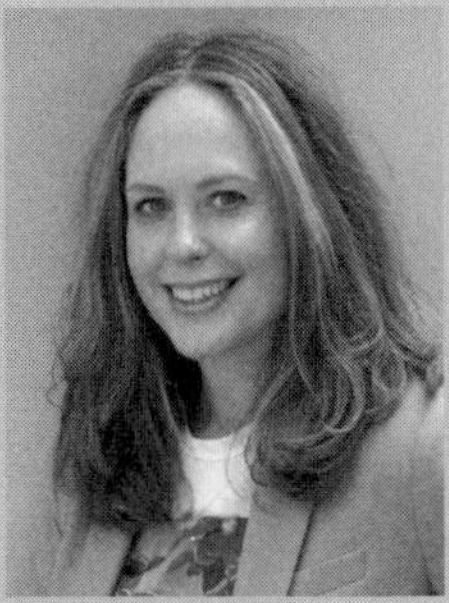

**Cara Wheatley-McGrain** is the founder of The Mindful Gut UK, a mindset and compassion coach, and an educational consultant. She is an expert patient who has lived with IBD and IBS for 20 years.

Following a hospitalization that resulted in her almost losing her colon, Cara resolved to develop a more mindful and empowered relationship with her gut. She has spent the last two decades cultivating an authentic whole-life approach to mindful, compassionate and intuitive gut care – and is now dedicated to sharing this powerful message of embodied self-care and holistic healing with those who are experiencing both short- and long-term symptoms of incurable IBS and IBD. Cara offers workshops to inspire people to learn to love and listen to their gut, and to raise awareness of the connection between good gut health and mental health.

Cara lives with her husband, David, and pup, Isla Mae. She has a family allotment and can be found there in her wellies most weekends.

**The Mindful Gut UK**

**@mindfulgutuk**

**The Mindful Gut UK**

**www.carawheatleymcgrain.com**